PREGNANCY *and* PARENTING

after THIRTY-FIVE

A JOHNS HOPKINS PRESS
HEALTH BOOK

PREGNANCY *and* PARENTING *after* THIRTY-FIVE

Mid Life, New Life

MICHELE C. MOORE, M.D.
CAROLINE M. DE COSTA, M.D.

THE JOHNS HOPKINS UNIVERSITY PRESS

BALTIMORE

© 2006 Michele C. Moore, M.D., and Caroline M. de Costa, M.D.
All rights reserved. Published 2006
Printed in the United States of America on acid-free paper

9 8 7 6 5 4 3 2 1

The Johns Hopkins University Press
2715 North Charles Street
Baltimore, Maryland 21218-4363
www.press.jhu.edu

Library of Congress Cataloging-in-Publication Data

Moore, Michele.
  Pregnancy and parenting after thirty-five: mid life, new life / Michele C. Moore,
Caroline M. de Costa.
      p.   cm.
  Includes bibliographical references and index.
  ISBN 0-8018-8320-2 (hardcover : alk. paper)—ISBN 0-8018-8321-0 (pbk. : alk. paper)
  1. Pregnancy in middle age   2. Childbirth in middle age.   3. Middle-aged mothers.
  I. De Costa, Caroline, 1947–   II. Title.
    RG556.6.M66 2006
    618.2—dc22   2005018223

A catalog record for this book is available from the British Library.

Contents

Part Four   BIRTH

Part Five   AFTER THE BIRTH

Appendices

Acknowledgments

We wish to thank Dr. Jeanne Wiebenga for her expert critical reading of our manuscript, Dr. Bob Miller for sharing his expertise on ART, and Cairns Base Hospital Library and its staff for helping us in our research. Our agent, Sally Brady, has been an unending source of encouragement and help. Javed de Costa and Josie Valese have been always willing to help with the finer points of word processing and computer vagaries. We thank Jacqueline Wehmueller, our editor, who requested that we write this book.

Last, but far from least, we thank our families, for their forbearance as we disappeared behind piles of paper, and the patients whose experiences we bring to this work.

PREGNANCY *and* PARENTING

after THIRTY-FIVE

Introduction

⁓

As you have probably discovered, there are many books about the physical changes of pregnancy, the normal growth of the baby, the search for a birth attendant, whether that person should be a doctor or a midwife, what happens in normal labor, and how to care for a newborn baby. However, few of these books speak authoritatively on these topics as they relate to a woman experiencing a pregnancy at a later time in her reproductive years. Those that do tend to be highly subjective and may be politically biased. This is OK; most people have a very personal viewpoint of childbirth, usually based on their own experience. But, there are many different ways of looking at the subject, and it is important for women over 35 to have the particular medical facts that apply to them.

The authors of this book are women and doctors, with a combined experience of over fifty years of caring for women; we are also mothers ourselves, and we feel very strongly that all women have the right to be informed, not only about how pregnancy and childbirth usually and normally proceed, but also about what can go wrong, and why, and what can be done about it. In this book we have tried to present this information in an unbiased way, so that each woman can make the best-informed choices for herself and her baby.

TRENDS IN LATER-LIFE PREGNANCIES

Everyone who reads a newspaper knows that many women—single or wed, in committed or casual relationships, for career or personal reasons—are deferring pregnancy until their later reproductive years. The median age of childbearing women in Massachusetts is now 30 years, whereas it was around 25 just twenty years ago. The U.S. Census shows that childlessness has doubled in the past twenty years and that one in every five women, or 20 percent, in the age group 40 to 45 has never had a child. For women 40 and younger who have professional training or graduate degrees, the figure is 47 percent. Economist Sylvia Hewlett, in her recent book *Creating a Life: Professional Women and the Quest for Children*, described a group of nearly 2,000 "high-achieving" women in business, law, and medicine and found that 42 percent were still childless after the age of 40; in the higher-paid echelons, the figure was closer to 50 percent. As Hewlett explains, and we will be discussing, not all of these women were childless by choice; but certainly most of them initially deferred their plans and hopes for children because they were pursuing career paths in competition with men, for whom having a family is not a hindrance to advancement in their jobs.

In the year 2000 in the United States, 546,674 women over age 35 had their first child. Successful intentionally deferred pregnancies are often popularly viewed as the typical "pregnancy after 35," but there are many other patterns of later pregnancy. Some women had children at a younger age and then decide for a variety of reasons to have one or more children later in life. Perhaps a woman who has been widowed or divorced remarries or re-partners and wants to have a child with her new spouse or partner; others may

Table 1.   Live Births in United States by Age of Mother and Birth Order

	All Ages	35–39	40–44	45–49	50–54
First baby	1,622,404 (40%)	100,334 (2.5%)	18,959 (0.5%)	1,053 (0.026%)	84 (0.002%)
Third baby	676,597 (17%)	106,281 (2.6%)	18,748 (0.46%)	725 (0.018%)	42 (0.001%)
Fifth baby	95,200 (2.3%)	22,208 (0.5%)	6,160 (0.15%)	306 (0.007%)	12 (0.0003%)
Eighth baby or beyond	18,342 (0.45%)	6,991 (0.17%)	3,953 (0.097%)	403 (0.0099%)	18 (0.0004%)
Total	4,058,814 (100%)	452,057 (11%)	90,013 (2.2%)	4,349 (0.1%)	255 (0.006%)

Source: Data from 2002 National Vital Statistics Report.

always have wanted a large family and so continue bearing children well into their forties; some women may find themselves unintentionally pregnant and decide to carry on with the pregnancy; some infertile women, because of the time and money involved in infertility treatment, are well into their later childbearing years before they successfully conceive. There are many reasons for later childbearing; the basic facts may be similar among different women, but the nuances are unique to each situation.

A Few Words about Medical Interventions in Childbirth

Much of the available literature on pregnancy deals with what has become known as "natural" childbirth and campaigns for minimal intervention during pregnancy and labor. It advocates avoiding epidurals and other forms of pain management, espouses the superiority of home births with midwives in attendance, and discourages use of Cesarean section delivery. Its arguments are often highly emotional and view "natural" childbirth as sacrosanct. This mindset is essentially a reaction to what we freely admit was excessive use of medical interventions in the processes of childbirth, a trend which reached its height in the 1980s. Most of these interventions were devised by doctors seeking to decrease death or damage to women and their babies in the course of pregnancy and birth. The interventions sometimes involved technologies that were new and, like many new things, had not yet revealed their limitations.

Certainly, the chances of a mother or baby dying during pregnancy or childbirth are now very much less than they were as recently as 1970, and most babies are now born alive and healthy. This happy situation is partly due to advances in obstetric care of mothers and in pediatric care of newborn babies, but it is also because women have become healthier, and a healthy mother is the best starting point for a healthy pregnancy outcome.

The campaign for less medical intervention and more involvement of women in decisions about their health care during pregnancy has been good in that it has led to the questioning of much dogma about obstetric care (for example, the necessity of shaves, enemas, and masks; the routine use of episiotomies and stirrups for normal births), and the movement has given many women a greater sense of control over what happens to them during pregnancy and labor. However, in our view this campaign has sometimes gone too far. In some instances, women are presented with rigid views of what constitutes femininity and its association with childbirth, with no allowance for individual circumstances. Women can end up feeling that the process of labor is a challenge at which they will either succeed or fail. This is both factually incorrect and morally wrong: there are many different ways of approaching pregnancy and childbirth, some of them medical, some not. Each woman is an individual, and her individual needs and preferences must be honored.

In most developed countries in the twenty-first century, birth, even for those desiring minimal intervention, still involves some contact with the medical and paramedical professions, and most babies are born in hospitals. The rationale behind hospital birth is that there need be no intervention if all is going well, but all the bells and whistles of modern medicine are near at hand, with the expert personnel to employ them, should a problem arise. Some people believe that home birth with the possibility of transfer to a hospital is as safe an option for mother and baby as hospital birth, and the example of Holland is often used. Holland is small in area and the population is densely clustered in urban areas. Home birth is a popular and relatively safe option there (about 30 percent of women choose it) at least partly because of very quick transit from home to the hospital for women experiencing any problems during birth. In larger countries such as the United States, Canada, and Australia, access to well-equipped hospitals is not usually as rapid and straightforward, so home birth is a less safe option for mothers, and particularly for babies.

The existence of modern technology does not negate the fact that significant risks to mothers and babies do still exist. Today in the United States, 20 to 24 percent of babies are born by Cesarean section, and the choice of this delivery method is usually made because of unacceptable risk to the mother or the baby if the pregnancy or labor is allowed to continue. Another 5 to 10 percent of first babies are born with the assistance of forceps or the vacuum extractor, for similar reasons. The advantage of modern medical technology is that the risks to mother and baby can generally be detected early or anticipated. When we know about risks in advance, it is far easier to take the appropriate steps to eliminate or minimize them. Many tests are available to women during pregnancy and labor, and some of these are especially relevant for the older mother. Other tests are routinely recommended for babies just after birth. These tests are well researched, supported by evidence in the medical literature, and offered because they provide protection and improved outcomes for mother and baby.

It has become widely accepted that pregnant women should have choices about how, where, and when they give birth, and we heartily concur. Most pregnancies proceed completely without significant complications, as do most labors and births, with the longed-for outcome of a healthy baby and delighted parents. However, it is only after the event that a birth can be judged to have been completely normal: pregnancy and birth do have the potential for going suddenly and dramatically wrong. If this happens, the presence of experienced obstetricians and midwives and other birth personnel can literally be lifesaving for a woman or baby. We therefore recommend that you carefully consider the issue of your baby's safety, and choose where you wish the birth to occur well before your expected due date. There is no socially or politically correct way to have a baby; there is only the best way *for you*. If medical intervention is necessary for your baby to be born healthy, then so be it. If childbirth were entirely left to "Nature," many mothers and babies would, quite "naturally," die—as they did in the past. That this was a frequent occurrence is borne out by meandering through old graveyards and reading the headstones.

Words like "normal," "natural," and "succeed" in the context of childbirth are often used with judgmental and emotionally motivated implications. Women sometimes tell us that they feel that they have "failed" at childbirth, even when they have birthed a beautiful and healthy baby, because their experience was more painful, difficult, or just plain different from what they had been led to expect and because they had accepted medical intervention. This altogether unjustified reaction is of particular concern when these feelings of inadequacy interfere with a mother's happy bonding with her baby. It was for this reason that we wrote our previous book, *Cesarean Section: Understanding and Celebrating Your Baby's Birth*—so that women who had already undergone or who might have C-sections would be well informed about the procedure. We have been similarly motivated in writing this book.

We are not apologists for the medical profession; indeed, many of our more conservative colleagues feel that our writing is too radical. We have been told that we should not so clearly describe some of the possible problems and solutions attendant on birth, that we risk exposing doctors to litigation. We think that reticence on these subjects would be a disservice to the women we write for. Medical intervention in pregnancy or childbirth should occur only after a thorough explanation and discussion with the woman and her partner about why it is being suggested; we know, however, that situations arise in pregnancy and childbirth that necessitate urgent decisions. Because of these possibilities, we believe that having access to information well in advance is desirable for every woman, but especially for women having babies in their later reproductive years, which is usually accepted to be 35 and over. This information is also necessary for women just *thinking* of pregnancy at this stage in their lives. They have choices that were not available to previous generations.

CHALLENGES FOR THE OLDER MOTHER

For the woman over 35, having a baby has particular challenges: emotional, social, and medical. Some of the medical conditions that are more prevalent in older women can complicate pregnancy, and there are greater risks of certain abnormalities in the baby. We are all a bit less adaptable as we get older, and it becomes more difficult to make the radical changes in lifestyle that come with having a baby. The constraints placed on career and financial circumstances may loom large. Many of these factors apply even when a woman has had children at a younger age; imagine the financial and social strains of simultaneously having a new baby and a child in college (we'll introduce you to several women in this situation).

Even when the expectant mother is in her forties, pregnancy and childbirth usually proceed normally, are trouble-free, and lead to the spontaneous vaginal delivery of a healthy baby. But it would be folly to ignore the fact that, statistically, older women are more likely to miscarry in early pregnancy, to have certain complications of pregnancy, and to deliver their babies via Cesarean section or with some other form of operative assistance. This is just how it is, and ignoring it will not change the facts.

Most women in this age group feel well in control of their lives and able to plan and execute their life decisions. It is important for them to realize that they may need to accept medical help—to conceive, to continue a healthy pregnancy, and to give birth to a healthy baby. We know about this first-hand, not just from the women for whom we've cared, but by our own experience. Michele gave birth to her first child, a vigorous boy, at the age of 35, by means of an emergency Cesarean section. This was totally at odds with her plans for this birth. Two and a half years later, she gave birth to her beautiful daughter by an elective C-section. The realities of being an older mother had sunk in, and she was grateful to be able to choose the planned C-section birth. Caroline is an example of women who have had children earlier in life and then decide later to have more. She has had seven children, the first at age 20 and the fifth at 33. For family reasons, eight years later, she and her husband decided on another pregnancy, and a wonderful son was born when she was 41. He was not the last, however, for at 44 she gave birth to a delightful daughter—her last child.

We also acknowledge that not all women who become pregnant in later life planned or welcome the situation, even though they may proceed with what becomes a much-wanted pregnancy and, after the birth, a most-cherished child. We will be discussing why women may feel conflicted about pregnancy.

About This Book

The book is divided into five sections: "Planning a Pregnancy," "Getting Pregnant," "Being Pregnant," "Birth," and "After the Birth." Each section first presents normal processes and procedures, then problems that may arise and how they may be dealt with. Obviously not all of this information will be relevant to every woman; using the table of contents and index, you can read what is relevant for you. We also provide a glossary of terms, a comprehensive list of resources, and several appendices containing specific data. We have not attempted to duplicate the general information about pregnancy and birth which is available in many excellent other books. Our aim is to deal only briefly with such general material but to provide the full spectrum of information needed by an older mother, from conception through to some often-difficult times of caring for children when you are the oldest mom at the PTA meeting. The book addresses such matters as preexisting medical conditions and how they may affect pregnancy, and difficulties with conception. Our approach is not intended to overemphasize problems but rather to deal with them in a realistic way for the woman who comes to pregnancy at a somewhat later age.

While we will occasionally refer to our own personal experiences, mostly we draw upon established knowledge and practice guidelines, up-to-date medical literature, and our clinical experience with patients. We have also included stories of women we have been privileged to care for. Names and details have been changed. We thank them all for sharing their stories with us.

Part One

PLANNING A PREGNANCY

———————————

Chapter 1

— ❧ —

Thinking about Pregnancy

Ideally, becoming a parent is a step considered with care. We all realize that this is not always the case, but as you are reading this book, you are clearly giving thought to this important decision. Many conditions in which we find ourselves can be changed, but once you discover you are pregnant, many processes in your body have already been set in motion.

There is nearly always a period of days or weeks between conception and when the woman becomes aware of being pregnant; this is true even for women who are trying to conceive and are very focused on what is happening inside them. The actual meeting of the egg and sperm—conception—happens about two weeks before the first missed period. Yes, it is true that some women experience changes in their bodies before they can otherwise have any clues of pregnancy (Michele was made nauseous by the smell of coffee, which she loves, almost immediately upon becoming pregnant), but most women remain uncertain until at least that first missed period.

Why does this matter? It matters because during the first three months of pregnancy (the first trimester) the fetus is the *most* vulnerable to outside influences that can be healthy or unhealthy for its development. Optimal maternal health is most important at this time, and the best way to create this good health is to start *before* you conceive. As a woman in your mid-thirties or older, you would be well advised to have a physical and a chat with your doctor before attempting conception, with the idea of identifying any particular challenges you might face during pregnancy—a previously undetected anemia or borderline high blood pressure, perhaps, or any one of a host of asymptomatic but potentially problematic conditions. Your doctor will probably want to check that you have regular, or fairly regular, periods; if you don't, then you may need referral to a fertility specialist to help with conception. A breast exam and mammogram, and a Pap smear, if you haven't had these tests recently, may be appropriate. These steps will allow you to address any important health issues before conceiving and thus to enter pregnancy at your best.

There are many things you can do to improve your health in the months before you become pregnant, all of which should continue into the early weeks of pregnancy and later. Obvious pieces of advice are: stop smoking, if you do smoke; discontinue that glass of wine or beer with dinner—or before, or after, or at any other time; watch your caffeine intake, keeping it at or below two cups of regular coffee or cola per day (see Appendix D for caffeine content of coffees, teas, colas, and chocolate). If you partake of "recreational" drugs, now is the time to stop . . . before conception.

If you need prescription medications, make an appointment to talk with your doctor about whether the drugs you are taking are safe during pregnancy, for you and the baby. The solution may be simple. For instance, Michele recently treated a woman who needed medication for her high blood pressure but who also wanted to have a baby. The woman was taking an ACE inhibitor, a very important and commonly used class of hypertension drug, but one that can cause problems with a developing baby's kidneys and urinary system. However, high blood pressure in pregnancy can also be dangerous, for baby and mother. A change to another class of blood pressure medication solved the problem for Michele's patient. We don't recommend that you stop your medications on your own; there is a good reason you are taking these drugs. With your doctor, come to a solution that will benefit the health of both you and your planned baby. In Appendices A and B you will find a listing of medications that may be harmful and ones that are generally safe to take when you are pregnant. Even if a drug is usually safe, a good rule of thumb is not to take it unless you truly need it for your health or you are truly uncomfortable and know that you will receive relief from it.

This would also be a good time to check and see if you are immune to rubella (German measles); if you are not and you are not yet pregnant, being immunized would be a good step (although you must then avoid pregnancy for at least two months). And, by "not yet pregnant" we mean that you have carefully used birth control and haven't even *tried* to get pregnant yet; you don't want inadvertently to take the rubella shot in early pregnancy.

What should you eat when you are planning to get pregnant? A basic answer in most circumstances would be lean protein, lots of fruits and vegetables, and whole grains. Included should be sources of the "good fats" from fish and seeds and nuts. Women embarking on pregnancy can especially benefit from folic acid. This vitamin of the B group helps prevent serious abnormalities of the brain and spinal cord in the developing baby. Because these problems develop early in the pregnancy, it is good to be aware of your folic acid intake before you begin trying to become pregnant. Folic acid is found in abundance in leafy greens, whole grains, oranges, cantaloupe, milk, bananas, and organic meats. You can hedge your bets by taking a multiple vitamin every day. Make sure it contains at least .4 mg (often expressed as 400 micrograms) of folic acid. *Do not take* the super-duper megavitamins offered at health food and nutrition stores, because they may very well have more vitamin A or C than is advisable for the developing baby. During your chat with your doctor, you could ask for a prescription for prenatal vitamins and calcium. These are compounded to supply exactly the micronutrients needed during pregnancy.

If you are very overweight, try to lose weight before you become pregnant. For many complicated reasons (some of which we will discuss later), being close to the normal body mass index can make it easier to become pregnant (see Appendix C). This doesn't mean you must go on a crash diet; it does mean eating in a healthy manner and eliminating the extra calories that many of us consume without even thinking about it. Before putting anything in your mouth, ask yourself, "Do I really *need* this? Is this high-quality nutrition that will give me vital nutrients, or is it just a high-fat, high-salt, or high-sugar treat? Am I eating because I'm hungry or because the food is there and eating is something to do?" Train yourself to eat only if you are hungry and to stop when you are no longer hungry. Eat from the high-quality food categories mentioned above. Remember that *health* is the aim, and your waistline is only one of the indices of health. Aim for a prepregnant waistline measurement of less than 35 inches.

One food to avoid is raw meat; raw meat can be contaminated with bacteria or parasites and can be a source of toxoplasmosis, a parasite that older children and adults tolerate well but that can cause birth defects in a developing baby. Also stay away from unpasteurized milk, and cheese or other products made from unpasteurized milk, which can be a source of the bacterial infection listeriosis, to which pregnant women have a heightened vulnerability.

Nearly everyone's health program should include exercise. If you have been a couch potato, prepregnancy is not the time to start weight lifting and marathon training, but a 30-minute walk twice daily would benefit you very much. Or you might enjoy a daily swim. Do *not* use a hot tub after your exercise, though; concerns have been raised that elevated maternal body temperatures in the first trimester of pregnancy can contribute to birth defects. If you are already very active, you can probably continue with your regular regime. However, if you are losing weight or if you have any questions, you should talk with your doctor and see if you need to modify your exercise program.

We have been asked if it is harmful to work with computers during early pregnancy. So far, this has not been shown to be the case, but do take routine breaks, simply to protect yourself from increased fatigue. Women who work in settings in which there are chemicals would be well advised to talk with the safety engineer at work and ask for "MSDS sheets" on all of the chemicals used. Take these fact sheets to your doctor and ask him or her to tell you if the chemicals in use might cause you or the fetus any problems. Again, doing this research and any self-protection before you become pregnant is best, but it is an important precaution and can still be helpful after conception. Doctors and nurses who work with anesthetic gases may need to take special precautions; discuss this with your own physician and your chief of service on the job. If you work with radiation, you should talk with your safety engineer and your own doctor and be certain what your levels of exposure and risks are.

If you are planning to get pregnant, you may as well cleanse your home of possible toxins at this time. It will easier to do it now than to try to accomplish it after the baby arrives (and soon thereafter starts crawling!). Most of the citrus-based cleaners are very good cleansers and have low toxicity potential. Your grandmother found vinegar to be a good cleanser and it still works. We are all better off not having in our homes any substance marked "harmful if ingested, inhaled, or spilled on the skin." Such products represent an accident waiting to happen.

We mentioned above that toxoplasmosis can contaminate raw meat, but the source of toxoplasmosis that people are most aware of is cat feces. No, you do not have to give the cat away. If possible, have someone else in the household empty the cat's litter box and clean it. If there is an unexpected mess that can't be left for someone else to clean up, use protective gloves and a mask during your exposure to the feces.

Mature women tend to be good at anticipating and planning ahead for the health of their babies. Gather information and approach issues in a proactive manner and you will minimize potential problems in your pregnancy. We hope that our advice proves helpful to you in having a healthy pregnancy and a healthy baby.

Chapter 2

————— ∾ —————

Making Choices about Work

Every mother is a working mother, but some also work outside their homes. If you are already established in your work, you may have the status and the accrued salary advances that come with experience; you may have seniority or the benefits of a unionized job; you may have accrued additional weeks of vacation and other advantages of long employment. Wherever you are in your work life, your employment situation and goals will have to be considered as you approach motherhood, whether for the first time or again.

Which Path to Take?

There are three basic questions you need to ask yourself before you bring your baby home—*long* before. They are:

- Do I want to work full time after I have my baby?
- Do I want to be a stay-at-home mother?
- Do I want to work, but with reduced hours and perhaps reduced responsibilities?

The answers may seem obvious to you, or you may find as you pose the questions that you are answering affirmatively to more than one option. Whatever the answers, arrangements regarding your employment need to be made well in advance of a baby's arrival.

If you wish to keep working full time, examine whether your current employment will be supportive of your family goals. If you are in a job that is not compatible with being a working mother, you may want to change employers or change jobs within your place of employment. It is hard enough to perform to your own standards in both motherhood and job without having unnecessary obstacles at work. Again, look at this situation before you are in the middle of juggling the two roles.

If you decide that you want to stay at home, either permanently or for a predetermined period of time, be as sure as you can of your decision. Realize that, although your baby will bring you incredible joy, you will have other needs that have until now been at least partially met at work. Adult conversation is one of these, and intellectual stimulation is another. Certainly, your partner will contribute in these areas, but it is a burden on a relationship to expect one person to fulfill all of your needs. Plan ahead to do some adult activities each week and to meet with other people. If you had a habit of lunching occasionally with other women, why should you stop? Even the stay-at-home mom needs a respite.

If you want to continue to work but would prefer to put in fewer hours and have less responsibility, explore the possibility of job sharing or look into part-time work. In the professions, job sharing is often a more viable option than a position that is truly part time. We have known husband and wife doctors who have shared a position, so that there was always a parent available to be at home with the children. Be creative, but above all, PLAN.

You and your spouse or legal partner need to learn your employers' policies on maternity and paternity leave. If your company employs more than 50 people, it is subject to the provisions of the federal Family and Medical Leave Act. You must have been employed by the company for at least one year and work at least 25 hours weekly. You can find out more about this at www.dol.gov/esa/whd/fmla.

See if any short-term disability plans at your job cover maternity leave. Many do not cover normal pregnancy and delivery, but most will cover you if you should have any complications of pregnancy. Some states have mandated plans. Ask what is available to you.

Find out ahead of time whether you will be required to use your medical and vacation leave before taking maternity or short-term leave. Janelle had to take medical leave every time she had a doctor's appointment, and she was dismayed to find she had no time left by the end of her pregnancy. It made a difference in her situation, because, working for a company with fewer than 50 employees, she then had to take unpaid time for her maternity leave. Had she realized her situation earlier, she would have arranged to do compensatory work for the hours taken to go to the doctor.

One way of juggling work and family that is increasingly popular is telecommuting. Andrea is a financial planner and used to go to her office in New York every day. Since she adopted Maire three years ago, she has been doing most of her work from her home computer and goes to the city only once a week. She now has two young children and says that this arrangement works beautifully for her family. Inez is a travel agent, and she convinced her agency to set her up at home as a remote office. This has worked so well that for three consecutive months, she has been the top-billing agent. Sometimes she needs a sitter to keep the children occupied and happy while she works at home, but she is just in the next room and able to be privy to all her children's milestones and aware of all their needs.

CHILD-CARE ASSISTANCE

Whether you plan to work full or part time, child care will be a vitally important part of your life and is another piece that should be arranged well before coming home with a baby in your arms. There are many options, and each one fits someone's needs. The possibilities include professional child-care centers, relatives, immediate family who work different shifts, in-home nannies, and other mothers who finance staying at home with their own children by sitting for other people's children. You can find a safe and comfortable arrangement with any of these solutions, but take nothing for granted and do your homework ahead of time.

You need to define your needs and criteria. The best way to do that is to make a checklist, so that you can rate each child-care option or practitioner that you evaluate (and that includes relatives). Among our concerns would be the following:

- Does the caregiver *like* children? Is she warm and caring?
- How does this person discipline children?

- Does this person have a plan for emergencies? Medical, staffing, etc.
- Does this person have credentials in early childhood development?
- Are you able to verify that this person has a good reputation?
- Does the environment support your child's development?
- Is the environment clean?
- What arrangements are made for children with minor communicable illness, for example, colds?
- What is the age of the youngest child accepted for care at this facility? And the oldest?
- Are babies and toddlers mixed in with older children?
- What are the hours of availability of this child care?
- Are you comfortable with this person on an intuitive level?

These questions will reveal important information that you will want to consider before choosing your child-care provider. Add your own concerns, and rank them by order of importance to you. The child-care provider will be a tremendously important part of your child's life and should be chosen with more care than you would give to buying a car or even a house.

Michele can attest to the importance of having a back up for your usual child care. Ill health or other problems can affect anyone, and such upsets of the routine seldom happen at convenient times. Michele's first-line child care was a woman trained as a preschool teacher who cared for children in her home. This woman became ill. Because Michele couldn't leave her patients high and dry, a back up was needed. Fortunately, across the road from Michele lived a retired schoolteacher who loved children and was happy to take over whenever she was needed. Not everyone has a wonderful neighbor like this, but a back-up child-care plan is absolutely necessary. Don't wait until you need it to put it in place.

FATIGUE

Another consideration for the older mom is that you will be tired much of the time. This is true for younger mothers, too, but they tend to bounce back more quickly than we do, so the fatigue is less cumulative for youthful mothers. You'll be getting less sleep, and the sleep you do get will most likely be disturbed. If you are breast-feeding, you'll be expending extra calories in producing milk, and the effect of this is that your body is working at three full-time jobs! It seems as though you no sooner get your baby to sleep through the night than you find yourself at the toilet-training stage and you're getting him up at night to avoid a wet bed. You just can't win, for a while.

Little children are bundles of energy, and keeping up with them is very draining. You can't put them on hold and you can't ignore what they are doing, because they may hurt themselves or destroy something. They seem to have an uncanny knack for detecting when you are distracted and using that moment to investigate for-bidden territory. Their charm ensures that you will hug and kiss them, but you will have to drag your weary bones to pick up what-ever they've dumped. This is exhausting.

Be realistic and accept that this *will* apply to you. While you are discussing names and decorating a nursery, discuss with your partner the sharing of household chores and child care. Accept all the help you can get; it will make the difference between fully enjoying moth-erhood and being too tired to properly participate in your own life.

Remember that what works for Susan down the street may not be what works for you. Make your own checklists to help you de-cide on your work options and the best child-care situation for you and your family.

Chapter 3

―――――― ❧ ――――――

Fathers, Partners, and Surrogate Fathers

Most women embarking on pregnancy in their later reproductive years will do so with the active involvement and support of a partner. And partners—male or female and with or without other children—will all have their own concerns about the pregnancy and the prospect of another person becoming a part of your relationship.

A man in his forties or older may approach fatherhood with a whole bucketful of concerns, even when the pregnancy has been planned and he is supportive and happy about it. On the one hand, he may be delighted with the prospect of having a child or children of his own to teach, play with, and generally parent. When an older father is well established and confident in his career and can take time out to play and just be with his child, the advantages to the child can be enormous. Jim, a family physician in his fifties, found he was able to transfer to part-time work in a group practice when his son Simon was born in his second marriage; Jim found himself spending—and enjoying—infinitely more time with Simon than he had with the two children of his first marriage, both born when Jim was just out of medical school and struggling to establish himself. On the other hand, an older father may be so busy with his work that he is simply unable to devote the time he would like to the ongoing tasks of parenthood. He may be anxious about the special responsibilities that attend raising a child at this stage of life. His worries may be financial if he'll be nearing retirement when this child will be in college and he's not sure he can adequately provide financing for both. He may be aware of a family history of heart disease and early morbidity and may feel that his future as a father is insecure. He may fear other illness and be worrying that he will sicken and die, leaving his child and partner while the child is still young. Many men are very reticent about expressing such fears; sympathetic understanding from their partners will help them deal with these concerns.

Most men, even in this age of two-income families, feel that they should be the main breadwinner. A man may see the advent of a child as a financial burden, especially if parenting will cause one of the partners to bring in less income. This feeling may cause guilt, but the guilt may not be expressed. The dynamics of the parenting relationship will benefit if all such concerns can be openly aired. The mother may also have such concerns.

When a child comes into a long-term relationship that until then has not involved children, there will inevitably be a startling and permanent change in the nature of that relationship. A daily existence previously centered on the two of you will be replaced by one directed at the needs of the demanding and squalling new arrival. While most men cope with this perfectly well, it is important to explore feelings and doubts about the anticipated changes well before the expected arrival date and to work through such issues as they arise later.

Men frequently worry that a baby will interfere with the sexual relationship of the parents, and this is a realistic concern because it certainly does happen. Again, discussing this concern openly will not make it disappear but may take away the sting. If the man doesn't express this concern, we suggest that the expectant mother bring it up; almost all men have some worry about this. Make a plan that is acceptable to both of you to express intimacy often and with regularity during the first year of your baby's life, even if this doesn't always include intercourse. Women: Find ways that are meaningful to him to assure him that he is still important to you even though so much of your time and energy is taken up by the baby. You are very aware of *your* turbulent emotions, but you may not be aware of *his*. His are not hormone-driven, as yours are, but they are equally real. The manifestations of your changing persona as you become a mother are easy to see; it isn't as obvious that he may be feeling that his familiar world is slipping away from under his feet even as he is also becoming a father. Between you, you become parents. Support each other through this.

The older father, like the older mother, may have less resilience and stamina to deal with sleep disruption and the emotional drains of being always "on call." He may be continuing to carry a heavy work schedule and may worry about deterioration in his work performance. Again, discuss the problem and find a solution that suits both of you.

An older father will be more likely to face certain health problems than will his younger counterparts. Sperm function does not decline with age in the same way that ovarian function declines, but erectile dysfunction becomes more common as men get older. This can certainly be a problem for older couples trying to conceive, when intercourse has to be tied in to a woman's fertile time. We will discuss this further in Chapter 5. Diabetes, heart disease, and high blood pressure may all interfere with sexual—and hence reproductive—function and may also cause a man anxiety about his ability to work and parent in coming years. Such health questions are best addressed well before embarking on pregnancy.

As you plan for your own work and for child care after the birth of your baby, you may want to consider the fact that many more fathers are staying home with their children and being the primary caregiver. It no longer raises eyebrows when a mother resumes her career and the father stays home with the baby. Some couples agree to alternate staying at home: Louise, a school principal, and Ted, a research librarian, took turns staying home for the first five years after Owen arrived in their lives. Ted was able to occupy short-term positions during Louise's school vacations, and he was the primary carer for the rest of the year. In the course of the book, we'll tell you about several couples who used variants of this method. There is no single ideal solution; the best one is simply the one that works best for you.

Fathers today are generally much more involved in the process of rearing children than they were a generation or two past. Most (but not all) fathers want to have a voice in all decisions regarding their children. Many want equal partnerships with the baby's mother, and are willing to shoulder equal division of the chores. Many people, women and men, have preconceived ideas of how child care should be organized. It can be hard to realize that different styles and approaches may be equally workable and beneficial. Prospective parents need to talk about these issues without either being judgmental of the other's ideas.

Single mothers will need to decide—if possible—how much a part of the child's life the biological father will be. Some biological fathers want to have a large part in their child's life, others to remain anonymous, and a few will be completely unaware of the child's existence. The mother will not necessarily have any choice in this. A woman who finds herself pregnant from a casual encounter, or who chooses to become pregnant in that way, or who conceives by artificial insemination from a donor or a sperm bank should not underestimate the importance of the male role in bringing up her child. This was a concern for Angela and her partner Vicky. Angela arranged sperm donation from a friend, Joel, who wanted to have a role in his child's life; so their daughter Mandy grew up with parenting from two mothers and her biological father, Joel. It was mostly harmonious. Another lesbian couple we know, who have a son and a daughter, both conceived through artificial insemination, make sure that their children have regular contact with the fathers of two heterosexual families they are good friends with. They believe that this contact benefits all concerned. The men in a child's life should be stable presences, so a longtime friend or a brother might make a better surrogate father than a boyfriend.

Fathers are also eligible for paternity leaves under the Family and Medical Leave Act if they work for a company employing more than 50 people, for more than 25 hours per week, and have been doing so for at least one year. Most paternity leaves are unpaid, so the family's need for income must be balanced with the need for time together. Most fathers want some time with their newly expanded family just after the baby is born; others may need to take more time when the mother returns to work. After a woman has had a Cesarean birth, the father's presence at home at least in the first week may be essential. Adopting a baby also entitles a father to family leave.

As for involvement during the birthing itself, not all partners, male or female, want to be present. The pendulum of custom has swung from completely excluding fathers from the labor room, which was the situation when we were medical students in the 1970s, to expecting that partners will be present at prenatal classes, prenatal doctor's visits, and throughout labor and birth. Although many people enjoy such participation, not all men—and not all women—have the emotional reserves or the personal traits needed to cope with it, even though they may be hugely supportive in other ways. If a husband or partner expresses reservations about his ability to help with the birth, these feelings should be taken seriously; a better choice as birth partner may be a sister or friend. Also, we have met a few women who felt more comfortable giving birth without their husband or partner present. If you feel this way, say so; don't feel pressured to accept a situation you are unhappy with. It's the long-term relationship together that is important for all of you as a family. Of course, if the partner does want to be included, this should be encouraged as much as possible.

Part Two

❧

GETTING PREGNANT

_____

Chapter 4

———— ∾ ————

Natural Conception

The number of births to women in the United States over age 35 declines with increasing age of the mothers (as illustrated in Table 1). This is not merely a matter of choice. The fact is that fertility declines with age, and the currently popular notion that it is easy to conceive after 35 is too rosy. In fact, fertility starts a slow decline at about the age of 27, and by 42, according to the Centers for Disease Control, a woman's chances of conceiving naturally and carrying to term a healthy baby are less than 10 percent. It is a disservice to you for us to try to sugarcoat these facts or for you to ignore them. Likewise, if you are having difficulty conceiving, do not think of it as your "fault." It is a biological phenomenon. And it does not mean that you cannot become a mother, in one way or another.

Barbra had had problems with her periods ever since she was a teenager; they were always heavy and painful, and she was diagnosed with endometriosis and fibroid tumors in her uterus. When Barbra was in her early twenties, she had an ectopic pregnancy. This was the only time she had become pregnant, although she had never been very careful about contraception. At age 38, she met Cory and they became inseparable. Much to her surprise, two years later she found that she was pregnant. She and Cory were ecstatic and began planning marriage and a family life together. However, at three and a half months she miscarried. The event created problems in their relationship.

Two months after the miscarriage, Cory and Barbra decided to go away for a weekend, to discuss whether they wanted to stay together and whether to try again for a pregnancy. They carefully went through all the decision-making flow sheets that they used in their jobs and found that the decision to stay together made sense in more than emotional ways . . . and, of course, they loved each other. Children seemed like a natural outflow of the love that they had for each other. So they tried for the next several months to conceive again, but nothing happened. They got married, and the week after their wedding they went for their first appointment at the fertility clinic.

Different circumstances prevailed for Marie, who had never had any problems with her menstrual cycles and is very healthy and fit. At 36 years old, she had been trying to conceive for a year but without success. More about Marie later.

Usual Ovulation

Why does fertility decline as we get older? In rather simple terms, the store of eggs (ova) that we have in our ovaries is present from the time we are born; as we grow older, the eggs age, too. Older eggs have less fertile characteristics, and this inhibits chances for conception. There are also fewer eggs available. At puberty there are about 250,000 potential eggs in a woman's ovaries. In each cycle, about thirty ova start to develop but only one ovum, or occasionally two, matures fully and is released in the process of ovulation. The rest are absorbed and disappear. So only about 400 eggs are ever ovulated in the course of a woman's reproductive years. By the time she reaches her forties most of her eggs have been ovulated or have simply never developed. Taking birth control pills does not delay this process; degeneration of eggs continues when a woman is on the pill. Also, as a woman gets older, the lining of her uterus is less hospitable to the implantation of a fertilized egg, because the hormones estrogen and progesterone, needed to maintain the lining, are less efficiently produced by the ovaries.

The ability to release eggs—ovulation—also decreases as a woman gets older. This decrease may be reflected in irregularity of the menses, and it is detectable in a rising FSH level, measured by a simple blood test. FSH (follicle stimulating hormone) is produced by the pituitary gland (which lies at the base of the brain). The pituitary gland is important in the control of ovulation. If the

FSH level is high, the pituitary is noting that ovulation has not occurred, and it is sending more FSH to tell one or the other of the two ovaries to develop and release an egg. When ovulation occurs, the estrogen hormone from that ovary feeds back to the pituitary gland, and the FSH level drops. If ovulation does not occur—because the supply of eggs or the efficiency of the ovary, or both, are declining—the FSH level stays high. Generally speaking, an FSH level higher than 15 is an indicator of impaired fertility.

There are now home tests available to see if you are ovulating. Besides answering that question, they calculate the best time to make love or attempt artificial insemination in order to conceive. First Response and ClearBlue Easy are two brand name tests, and some of the drugstore chains have their own brands. These tests measure the rise of the hormone LH (luteinizing hormone). Like FSH, LH is a pituitary hormone that is directly related to the process of ovulation, but it can be measured in urine. The LH level rises about 24 to 36 hours before ovulation.

Once ovulation has occurred, the egg remains able to be fertilized for about 12 hours. After it leaves the ovary the egg is picked up by the fimbriae, fringelike projections at the outer end of the Fallopian tube that waft the egg along inside the tube. Sperm can live healthily in a woman's body for about 24 to 36 hours after ejaculation, hanging around in the Fallopian tube, which they reach by passing through the cervix and up the inside of the uterus. Conception takes place in the outer third of the Fallopian tube, and then the fertilized egg travels down into the uterus and settles into a suitable spot in the prepared uterine lining. This journey takes about four days. So, the usual advice to those trying to achieve pregnancy is to have intercourse at least every second day around the time of ovulation, in order to be sure there are some fresh and viable sperm available to impregnate the egg when it is released.

INTERFERING CONDITIONS

Pelvic problems like endometriosis or fibroids can interfere with this usual process of conception, as they did in Barbra's case. Younger women with such conditions are usually advised to attempt conception for up to a year before consulting a fertility clinic; many will conceive during this time. For older women, most doctors would not suggest as long a trial period. Sometimes, the option of proceeding directly to assisted reproduction may be presented immediately. This will vary with your circumstances. It was certainly appropriate for Barbra, who, by the time she arrived for her first visit to the fertility clinic, was 41 with a known history of both endometriosis and fibroids.

If you are over 35 and you have not conceived after six months of trying, it is time to seek help—*if you want to.* Not everyone will feel that it is essential to pursue every high-tech possibility in order to have a baby. Some couples decide to pursue fulfillment through other interests and life goals, even electing to use contraception to avoid pregnancy altogether thereafter. Others follow a "let's not worry about it, but if it happens, it happens" approach. An increasing number of couples, and even singles, adopt children; and some people satisfy their urge for parenthood or further parenthood by being foster parents to children already born but in need of care. We discuss these options in Chapter 9.

Another reason for decreased fertility in older women is that a greater percentage of us suffer from chronic illnesses, such as diabetes and hypertension, and our compromised health diminishes our reproductive abilities. From the point of view of evolution and the perpetuation of the species, this makes sense. For twenty-first century women in developed countries, it seems less relevant, because we have the benefit of excellent health care during our pregnancies. Several common chronic diseases and other conditions that may affect an older mother's pregnancy are discussed in Chapters 6 and 7.

Timing Conception Attempts

If you are an older woman trying to conceive, you can't rely on passion alone to determine when you have sex. You will want to track your menstrual cycles and make sure that intercourse happens during your fertile time. This is natural family planning—but planning *for* conception this time. There are several ways to figure out when you are fertile: the calendar, basal temperature, and vaginal secretions. To be most accurate, you can use a combination of the three. Or, you can opt for technology and purchase one of the over-the-counter ovulation predictors previously mentioned. (If you already realize you are having trouble conceiving, your doctor can order a test of your progesterone level on day 21 of your cycle, also showing your prolactin level, which, if elevated, could be interfering with your ability to become pregnant.)

If you are very regular in your cycles, a calendar may be all you need. Ovulation typically occurs 14 days before the onset of bleeding—around day 14 in a 28-day cycle. When a woman is using this method of timing to prevent conception, she usually designates days 9 through 17 as the "unsafe days"; for you, having intercourse every other day during this window of time would increase your probability of conception.

Of course, not every woman has cycles of 28 days with clockwork regularity, even in her twenties. So, to calculate when you ovulate from a calendar record of your cycle you should subtract 14 days from the usual length of your cycles. In other words, if you have cycles of 35 days, you could expect to ovulate on day 21; if your cycles are 26 days long, ovulation would occur around day 12; and in cycles varying between 27 and 32 days, ovulation would fall somewhere between days 13 and 18.

Cycles that have become very irregular, especially in a woman in her forties, may be a sign of impending menopause, and the woman may be ovulating very infrequently or not at all. If this describes you, you should talk with your doctor as soon as you even consider the possibility of pregnancy for yourself.

The basal-temperature-tracking method involves taking your temperature just as soon as you wake up every morning and recording it on a chart. Just after ovulation, a woman's body temperature rises by a fraction of a degree and remains elevated for two or three days. This is her fertile period. It is best to buy a special basal-temperature thermometer, because you will be looking for a fraction of a degree of change in your temperature. Drugstores, family planning clinics, and sites on the Internet all sell these instruments. They are not expensive.

The "mucus method," called the Billings method, of determining fertility relies on alterations in the cervical mucus that are caused by the hormonal changes during your menstrual cycle. To use this method, you feel high up in your vagina, touching the noselike knob that is your cervix and the mucus secreted from the cervix. During the rest of your cycle, this mucus is thick and sticky; when you ovulate it becomes thinner and runny, resembling egg white. Obviously, it takes practice to detect these changes. You should record your observations of both mucus and temperature in order to adequately appreciate daily differences.

Jean, a patient of Caroline's, used the Billings method to calculate when she was ovulating. She called her partner, Phil, on his cell phone to tell him to come home early for impregnation. Phil is an architect, who happened to be on site — on the scaffolding of a church tower his firm was restoring. He just about fell off in his excitement to rush home — to the immense amusement of the other workers. Baby Isabel was the architecturally inspired creation who appeared nine months later.

This is a true story. Similar fictional situations have been the subject of several films. These are always comedies, but in real life, having sex by the manual is not always romantic and may strain your sense of humor after a while. Remaining aware of the best time for conception and then maintaining as much spontaneity as possible will help you both through this. This may be the time to try such things as whipped cream, flavored massage oils, and erotic music. It is also good to openly and honestly discuss at the beginning how long you will try for an unassisted conception before consulting a specialist, or deciding not to.

Other Impediments to Natural Conception

Although it may sound very obvious, it is also important that you actually have vaginal intercourse and that your partner ejaculate into your vagina. Both Caroline and Michele have been consulted by couples who were technically virginal, although they didn't realize it. The cause can be lack of knowledge about one's anatomy, shyness, or a style of religious upbringing that portrayed sex as dirty or forbidden. We have also seen occasional cases where a woman's hymen was unusually thick and where full intercourse had never occurred. In some women, pain experienced with initial intercourse, or fear of such pain, may bring about a spasm of the muscles around the vagina (vaginismus), making penetration difficult or impossible. In men, premature ejaculation or erectile dysfunction may mean that full intercourse with a depositing of sperm high in the vagina—the necessary conditions for natural conception—are not occurring. If you are experiencing one of these situations, please be aware that solutions are readily available, provided by competent and sympathetic people.

Some older women who desire children will have come to know themselves as women who love women, whether they are in a long-term partnership with another woman or not. There has been a shift in public opinion over the past twenty years, and with it has come a greater acceptance of lesbian couples and their right to bring up children. Sexual preference does not determine a woman's fitness for motherhood nor how well she rears her children.

Many lesbian women negotiate directly with a man who agrees to donate his sperm so that they can inseminate themselves, by the old "turkey baster" technique long used by heterosexual women as well. Sometimes they will have their partner deposit the semen in the vagina for them, so they are sharing the conception of the baby. Other lesbian women prefer to go to a clinic providing artificial insemination using donor sperm.

Clinics that perform artificial insemination have the advantage that the donor has been screened for sexually transmitted diseases and his personal and family health histories have been recorded and are maintained on file. He also contracts to practice safe sex during the times that he is donating sperm. These clinics may be expensive, so making thorough inquiries is a good idea. Women who use sperm from a known donor by private arrangement are well advised to be sure that he is generally healthy, practices safe sex, and is free of any sexually transmitted infections, and should make note of any inheritable diseases in his family history. Whenever donor sperm is used, family history will also let the child know in later life who is too close a relation for marriage.

Any kind of artificial insemination should be carried out at the time of ovulation (determined by the methods described above) and should use fresh sperm, no more than 2 hours old. If you are using the do-it-yourself method, the man should ejaculate into a clean container. You should draw the semen from the container using a 5-cc hypodermic syringe from which you have removed and safely discarded the needle. Then insert the syringe into the vagina until it touches the cervix. You then squirt out the semen and hope it will be mission accomplished. If you have had an orgasm immediately prior to insemination, the sperm may be able to pass through the cervix more easily, so your partner can be a big help and feel lovingly part of the process.

All of the caveats about fertility apply equally to lesbian women, so decide early how long you want to try and whether you want to use assisted reproductive technology if you do not conceive.

It may seem like we are pouring cold water on your dreams of motherhood, but a book that did not tell you how it really is would leave you without the tools to make wise and well-grounded decisions. This subject is, after all, something that we understand very well, both as doctors and as mothers.

In the following chapters, we will discuss the various methods of assisted reproduction. There is a brave new world of high-tech ways of becoming pregnant. We will acquaint you with the various techniques and explain when they may be helpful and when they may not. We will also discuss other means of becoming a mother, what might be called "socially assisted" motherhood. These include adoption, surrogacy, and foster parenting. All of these are legitimate and rewarding paths to motherhood which no book about motherhood in a population of women with decreased fertility should ignore.

Chapter 5

———— ∾ ————

Assistance with Conception

If you have been trying to conceive for six months without success, it may be appropriate to visit your doctor for help in finding out what's preventing conception. The factors that decrease fertility fall into three main groups: First, problems associated with ovulation—you must produce eggs (ova) in order to conceive. Second, what is referred to as male factor infertility or subfertility—the man's sperm count and the normalcy of the sperm produced and their ability to get from where they are produced (in the testes) to where they will fertilize the egg (in one of the woman's Fallopian tubes). In an older man erectile dysfunction may also be a consideration. Third, there may be mechanical problems in the woman—such as blocked Fallopian tubes, endometriosis, or fibroids—that are interfering with the normal process of conception.

What Happens Next?

If you have decided to investigate a lack of success in conceiving, what can you expect? Initially, a full history of your health should be taken if it is not already known to the doctor. Family physicians and internists are best at history taking. If not already in your record, a full sexual history will be needed. Don't be embarrassed—these questions are not prurient; they relate directly to your wish to conceive. You will be asked questions like the following: Do you and your partner have full vaginal intercourse? How often? Is your cycle regular? Do you keep a menstrual calendar (we recommend that you do so in advance of the appointment and bring it along)? Do you plan intercourse to happen during your fertile time? Does your partner have any difficulty with erection or ejaculation? Has your partner fathered any children (or pregnancies that did not go to full term)? Has either of you had any sexually transmitted infections? Have you ever been pregnant? In asking these questions your doctor is looking for any possible barriers to your becoming pregnant, especially those that are readily treatable.

You should also have a general physical, which will include a check of your abdomen and likely an internal exam, unless you have recently had one. Your doctor may also suggest testing your thyroid gland and screening for diabetes; both of these require blood tests at a lab.

Some hormone levels may be tested at this stage. The progesterone level on day 21 of your cycle is commonly measured (counting

Causes of Infertility

In Females

Declining egg quality
Early menopausal changes
Endometriosis
Pelvic inflammatory disease (PID)
Fibroids
Tubal abnormalities
Anovulatory cycles for any reason
Polycystic ovary disease

In Males

Low sperm count or abnormal sperm
Erectile dysfunction

In Females and Males

Hormonal abnormalities
   (diabetes, thyroid disease)
Medications
Cancer treatment
   (chemotherapy, radiation)

the first day of your period as day 1; the test day may be adjusted slightly by your doctor to reflect your cycles). Progesterone is a hormone produced by the ovaries; the level of progesterone should be elevated if you have ovulated in that cycle. Your prolactin level may also be measured. Prolactin, a pituitary hormone, is responsible for milk production when a woman is lactating, and it inhibits ovulation. Sometimes even without lactation there can be excessive production of prolactin, and this abnormal level prevents ovulation. Certain prescription medications can elevate your prolactin level. Very occasionally, the prolactin level may be elevated because a tumor of the pituitary gland is producing prolactin. Whatever the cause, raised prolactin levels are usually managed by drug treatment under the direction of an endocrinologist, rather than by surgery.

Also usual at this point is a pelvic ultrasound, to look at the outline of the uterus and ovaries and see whether there are any fibroids or polyps inside the uterus or cysts on an ovary and to check the size of the ovaries generally. An ultrasound will give some idea of how many potential eggs are still present in the ovaries and can pick up on some mechanical problems that might need to be dealt with.

The next step may be a check of your Fallopian tubes, and for this you will be referred to a gynecologist, if you haven't seen one already. There are a number of ways of checking the Fallopian tubes. One is laparoscopy, which we will describe. This procedure is less common now in the United States for older women who are not conceiving naturally, because they are now more readily recommended for assisted reproductive technology (ART, discussed in the next chapter). What happens in a laparoscopy? Under a general anesthetic a fiber-optic tube, the laparoscope, is inserted into your abdomen through a small incision. There is a tiny camera on the end of the laparoscope, and with it the doctor can look at the uterus, tubes, ovaries, and other organs within the pelvis, and test whether the Fallopian tubes are open. Some blue dye may be passed through your cervix, and a video screen will show whether or not the dye appears in the Fallopian tubes.

A laparoscopy is surgery, and there are risks (see box below), however, it will definitely give good information about your pelvic anatomy and function. Your surgeon will be able to check that your ovaries and the external surfaces of the tubes and uterus appear normal, to discover any adhesions (scarring) from previous surgeries or infections, and to see whether any endometriosis is present.

Marie, the healthy 36-year-old mentioned in the previous chapter, had a laparoscopy after all other exams and tests had failed to explain why she had been unable to get pregnant. The laparoscopy showed some adhesions around her right Fallopian tube from her appendectomy, but otherwise her uterus, tubes, and ovaries all appeared normal. During the laparoscopy, the surgeon went in and divided the adhesions. That procedure may have done the trick, because two months after the surgery she was happily pregnant.

In fact, statistically, there is a small increase in pregnancy rates 2 to 4 months following laparoscopy, even when no specific treatment is performed.

There are a couple of other ways to test the patency (openness) of the Fallopian tubes. One is a hysterosalpingogram, an x-ray of the uterus and tubes in which dye that is opaque to x-rays is introduced through the cervix and a series of radiographic pictures is taken, following the progress of the dye through the tubes. You don't need an anesthetic for this procedure, but it is uncomfortable,

---

RISKS OF LAPAROSCOPIC SURGERY

- Anesthesia risks: pneumonia, allergy to anesthetic drugs, very rarely death
- Bleeding necessitating opening the abdomen with a larger incision (laparotomy) to stop the bleeding
- Damage to bowel or bladder from instruments, requiring laparotomy for repair
- Postsurgical infection in the abdomen or bladder, requiring antibiotics
- Thrombosis (clot) in the leg veins with possible spread to the lungs

and some sedation or pain killer prior to the procedure is recommended. A hysterosalpingogram may be done in conjunction with an inspection of the inside of your uterus with a hysteroscopy (as distinct from the laparoscopy, which looks at the outside of the uterus). A hysteroscopy does not require an incision; it uses a fiberoptic tube threaded up the vagina and through the cervix. With a hysteroscope, your doctor can tell whether there are any fibroids or polyps intruding on the inside of the womb, sometimes removing small ones, and can see whether the inner openings of your Fallopian tubes—the ostia—appear normal.

An ultrasonogram is another way to detect polyps and fibroids that may be fully or partially blocking your tubes. The quality of the ultrasound picture can sometimes be improved by putting saline solution into the uterus; then it is called a contrast ultrasonogram. Ultrasound can also give a good idea of the size and functioning of a woman's ovaries, and therefore provide an indication of her chances of conceiving naturally or her likely response to infertility treatments using her own eggs (discussed in the next chapter). Quite often, ultrasound imaging is the main form of investigation used in older women trying to conceive, and it is done to help decide whether assisted reproductive technology is appropriate, and if so, what approach should be used.

Because some of these investigative procedures come with certain risks to you, before proceeding with them your family doctor or gynecologist should arrange for your partner to be checked. The first step usually is a seminal analysis, referred to—not completely accurately—as a "sperm count." If the analysis detects problems, or if you or he is aware of difficulties with his sexual functioning, he will need to have a chat with a physician. As we've mentioned already, either erectile dysfunction, more common in older men, or premature ejaculation can interfere with a woman's achieving pregnancy. Neither condition necessarily interferes with a sexual relationship otherwise, so they may not warrant treatment; but if you are trying to get pregnant, they can be significant, and treatments do exist. We should also say that the fact that a man has conceived a child in a previous relationship is not necessarily evidence that he is still fertile, for a number of reasons. He may have developed a varicocele, a collection of varicose veins in the scrotum. Or he may have had an infection, such as gonorrhea or trichomonas, that has either blocked the vas (the tube leading from the testis to the penis) or interfered with the quality of the sperm. Ejaculation of fluid may still be occurring, because some of the seminal fluid comes from the prostate and the seminal vesicles, which lie much closer to the start of the urethra, the canal that lies in the center of the penis and through which urine and seminal fluid pass.

For seminal analysis, the best specimen of semen is produced after three to four days abstinence from sexual activity. Arrangements need to be made for testing of the specimen while it is fresh; it should be examined in the lab within two hours, preferably. The man should produce the semen sample by masturbation, because commencing intercourse and then withdrawing may result in contamination of the sample by the woman's vaginal secretions. For clients who live far from the lab many clinics have facilities on site where the sample can be generated in privacy.

Seminal fluid analysis assesses more than the number of sperm. Normal figures for a sample are shown below.

- Volume: should be greater than 2.5 cc
- Sperm count: should be greater than 20 million per cc
- Motility: more than 50% of the sperm should be actively swimming
- Morphology (normal appearance): no more than 15% should be abnormal

If one or more of these factors is abnormal, the test should be repeated. Often the second test is normal. If an abnormality is detected in any of your or your partner's tests, then treatment needs to be considered. If the problem is male factor infertility, you may wish to attempt artificial insemination (ICSI, intracytoplasmic sperm injection, discussed in next chapter); sperm may be insufficiently active or antisperm antibodies may be present.

If insufficient ovulation is detected, drugs can be used to produce natural conception or to lower prolactin levels or as part of assisted reproduction treatment (next chapter). If there is tubal obstruction (for example, scarring due to endometriosis or previous infection, or fibroids, or some other cause) then ART may be needed. Surgery to open the tubes does not have a great record of success in these circumstances and has largely been abandoned in favor of ART.

Women with elevated prolactin levels will need the assistance of an endocrinologist or reproductive medicine specialist. Treatment will likely include medication, such as bromocriptine or cabergoline. Such medications tend to be effective very quickly in bringing about ovulation, with conception possible within a couple of cycles. Clomiphene is another medication that can help stimulate ovulation in women. It acts on the pituitary gland and on the part of the brain controlling the pituitary gland (the hypothalamus) to raise the levels of FSH and LH thereby effecting ovulation. Side effects of clomiphene include hot flashes, and sometimes cysts can develop rapidly on the ovaries, causing lower abdominal pain. Generally a low dose is given at first, and the woman is monitored with measurements of her progesterone level on day 21, to see whether ovulation is occurring. The dose can then be gradually increased. Another effect of clomiphene is the release of more than one egg; consequently, twins are more common in women who use this treatment. Obviously, clomiphene and the other drugs used to bring about ovulation can work only if there are sufficient high-quality eggs in the ovaries to be ovulated.

A decision to use any conception assisting drug or ART, or to use donor eggs, needs to be made in close consultation with a gynecologist or reproductive medicine specialist, after careful consideration of your age, medical history, hormone measurements, and ultrasound results. If nothing abnormal is found during your general investigations and laparoscopy, most gynecologists would recommend "hanging in there" for a few more months to see if conception happens naturally before proceeding to ART, although this depends on your age and circumstances.

It's also a good idea to talk through how much time, extraordinary effort, and expense you want to expend on trying to get pregnant, and to have in mind a definite point where you will stop. Be advised, however, that many a couple, having passed that endpoint and "given up," has some time later succeeded. Caroline's patient

Roma, a woman of 42, went through six cycles of in vitro fertiliza-tion to no avail. She decided to go back to art school. When she was 44, she thought she'd reached menopause, because her periods had stopped. Nope—she now has four-year-old twin girls conceived naturally!

REVERSAL OF FEMALE STERILIZATION

Changes in circumstances may cause a woman who has previously undergone a "sterilizing" procedure to think about having it re-versed so that she can attempt to become pregnant. Obviously, very often such a woman will be older than 35.

Sterilization of women and men is always done with the caution that it must be regarded as irreversible. In women sterilization is quite major surgery, requiring both general anesthesia and access to the inside of the abdomen. These days, the Fallopian tubes are most often closed off with clips (Filshie clips), which look like tiny clothes pins, or with rings of metal or plastic. Whatever method is used, the aim is to prevent the passage of eggs down the tubes from the ovaries and the progression of sperm up the tubes, so that "never the twain shall meet." Before a decision is made for steril-ization, most doctors and family planning clinics discuss the pro-cedure very fully with their patients, emphasizing its finality. And most women deciding for it believe that they will not change their minds about wanting more children no matter what . . . even if they should divorce or lose their partner or an existing child to illness or accident.

But, how we will feel under changed circumstances is not always predictable. Partners do sometimes move on, or die, and relation-ships break down and are replaced by new ones. And, sadly, even in developed countries, children die, not as uncommonly as you might suppose. It is impossible truly to predict how one will feel in such a situation. Some women who have lost a child find, after the initial grief and disbelief has passed, that they want to get pregnant again. This is not to replace the dead child but, as some women have expressed it to us, more like a tree or vine that has lost a branch but puts out new shoots. Simply because it takes time to have a first family, to go through the trauma of loss, and then to decide on trying to bear another child, many women in this position are likely to be in their later reproductive years. The following case stories illustrate issues that should be considered before reversing a sterilization.

M*ary was 32 when she agreed with her husband Sam that she should have a sterilization. Maybe Sam had been a bit keener than she was, but she had two healthy sons. Two years later, Sam announced that he was divorcing her and moving in with another woman. Four emotionally turbulent years later, at age 38, Mary met Tony and began to experience the love and support she deserved. Tony had never had children, and he came from an ethnic background that favors large families.*

Mary went for a chat with her gynecologist, who had carried out the laparoscopic application of clips for her. Mary was having regular cycles and was otherwise healthy. Her GYN recommended testing for ovulation; her day 21 progesterone level was fine. Tony had a seminal analysis done, and it was pronounced perfectly normal. So Mary underwent open-abdominal surgery, a laparotomy in which a bikini cut was made low on her abdomen, and a microsurgical reanastomosis (reconnection) was performed. Each clip was carefully cut out, along with the underlying segment of tube. Then the two ends of the tube were joined with stitches as fine as spider's web, so that the canal of the tube was restored. She was advised by her surgeon to wait for two months before trying to conceive. When she did try, she became pregnant right away. She has since gone on to have three sons with Tony, brothers to her two older boys. (Now she thinks it's Tony's turn for surgery.)

To do the reanastomosis, Mary chose a surgeon with a good reputation who frequently performs this particular operation. She was lucky to have gone into the procedure with healthy tubes and to be very fertile. In good hands and with fortunate conditions, the figures for successful pregnancy after reanastomosis when clips have been used are around 95 percent. The figures are not so good if there are adhesions (scarring) from previous surgery or if there has been any kind of infection.

Cecelia's daughter died when she was just two years old, from a rare childhood cancer. Cecelia had twice given birth by C-section and had a sterilization done during the second surgical delivery. Rather than applying clips to her Fallopian tubes, the surgeon had cut away a portion of each tube. Cecelia underwent a reanastomosis, but her surgeon warned her that the resulting length of tube was shorter than normal. Cecelia did become pregnant, but it was an ectopic pregnancy—a recognized possibility after reversal surgeries. The whole tube had to be removed in an urgent open-abdominal operation. After much consideration Cecelia decided to follow her doctor's recommendation to try ART, and after two cycles of treatment she was pregnant. A very anxious eight months followed until another daughter was born, a little early but well, by a third C-section.

IMPORTANT POINTS ABOUT REVERSAL OF FEMALE STERILIZATION

- Reversing sterilization is major surgery.
- Cost may be an issue.
- If simple clips or rings were used, results are better, because less tube has been destroyed. Where a larger amount of tube was removed or where tubes were diathermied (burnt)—not commonly done now—results are much poorer.
- Ectopic pregnancy is more frequent after a reversal.
- Successful pregnancy also depends on the overall fertility of both partners.
- The best outcomes result when the surgeon has had extensive experience doing this procedure.
- If you anticipate complications or if the procedure does not work, ART may be a better option.

Reversal of Male Sterilization (Vasectomy)

When the main barrier to pregnancy is that the male partner has had a vasectomy, reversal can be attempted. In the same way as reanastomosis is done for women, the separated ends of the vas, the tube which carries sperm from the testis to the outside world, are rejoined. This rejoining leads to successful pregnancy in around 50 to 70 percent of cases if there are no other barriers to conception. Sometimes, although the anatomy is restored, since the vasectomy there have been changes in the quality of the sperm which decrease the possibility that conception will occur naturally. Increasingly, artificial insemination or assisted reproductive technology is being used for men in this situation, with good results.

Chapter 6

——— ❧ ———

Assisted Reproductive Technology

ART, assisted reproductive technology, includes all procedures and treatments that involve the handling of human eggs and sperm and embryos for the purpose of establishing a pregnancy. It does not include artificial insemination, in which sperm either from a woman's partner or from a donor is introduced into the uterus so that conception can occur in the usual way.

Here are some terms you will need to know to follow this discussion:

fertilization: the penetration of the egg by a single sperm and the fusion of the genetic material of the two to form a *zygote* with the potential to develop into a baby

in vitro fertilization, IVF: the fertilization of an egg by a sperm outside of the mother's body, in the laboratory (popularly known as test-tube babies). The egg may be the woman's own or a donor's, and the sperm may come from her partner or a donor.

gamete: a cell that contains the genetic material from one parent; a sperm or an egg (either immature—oocyte—or fully developed—ovum)

zygote: a fertilized egg; the single cell formed by the union of the sperm and the egg

embryo: the product of conception from the time of fertilization until eight weeks later

fetus: the product of conception from eight weeks until birth

clinical pregnancy: an early pregnancy diagnosed by measuring hormone levels in the woman's blood or seeing early signs of pregnancy (like a gestational sac) on ultrasound

live-birth delivery rate: the number of live babies born per 100 cycles of ART

oocyte donation: oocytes (immature eggs) donated by another woman

cryopreservation: the freezing and storage of eggs, sperm, or embryos to allow later attempts at ART or because the person concerned will be undergoing surgery or treatment that might result in sterility and wishes to keep reproductive opportunities open

intracytoplasmic sperm injection, ICSI: the injection of a single sperm inside an egg that is ready to be fertilized. This is a very delicate technique. A sperm specimen may be obtained from a man with a low sperm count, by masturbation or by a clinical procedure. In men who have an obstructed vas (the tube bringing sperm from the testis), a needle may be directed into the testis to draw out the sperm. This procedure, TESA (testicular sperm aspiration), is done with a local anesthetic. Or, a piece of the sperm-producing tissue may be removed from the testis rather than sperm themselves. In another variant, MESA (microscopic epididymal sperm aspiration), sperm are aspirated from the epididymis, a coiled structure connecting the testis to the vas. ICSI, available for about twelve years, has been very successful in achieving pregnancy for couples with male factor subfertility—so much so that it is being used even when the man's sperm count is apparently normal but the couple for no obvious reason are not getting pregnant.

THE PROCESS

We generally talk about ART as occurring in cycles. A cycle of ART begins with the stimulation of the woman's ovaries to produce eggs (oocytes). Commercially produced gonadotrophin (ovary-stimulating) hormones are used in higher than usual doses to stimulate "super-ovulation," or more eggs than would normally be produced and brought to maturity in one cycle. The development of these oocytes is monitored by ultrasound until they are ready to be released from the ovary (ovulation). Ultrasound checks are performed at least three or four times in the early part of the cycle, sometimes every day, along with measurements of estrogen and other hormones. Maturation of the oocytes is then brought about by giving a synthetic form of luteinizing hormone, a pituitary hormone related to ovulation. At this point, the eggs are "harvested" using a long needle passed through the upper part of the vagina with ultrasound guidance. This egg retrieval is done under light sedation in a clinic or hospital.

This is the process embarked upon by Barbra, as she turned to ART after a miscarriage, a long history of endometriosis and fibroid tumors, and an early ectopic pregnancy.

Barbra hadn't realized that her endometriosis would make conception and pregnancy so challenging. She and Cory decided to try ART, but only after a long, hard look at their finances: their insurance didn't cover any type of infertility treatment, let alone ART. Fortunately, they had both been employed full time at good wages for all of their adult lives, and they'd been thrifty, saving systematically. They decided that they could afford to try ART for three cycles. If they were not pregnant at the end of that time, then they would need to reconsider.

Barbra took some accrued vacation time for her first cycle of treatment and was glad she had done so. Most of the time, because of the hormones, she felt as though she had mega-PMS: she had nausea, tender breasts, and headaches, and was on an emotional roller coaster. She was very grateful that she had support not only from Cory but also from the experienced nurses and counselor at the clinic. "Without them, I think I'd have lost my mind," she said. Cory was good about going with her for the ultrasounds and egg harvesting, but he was as nervous as a cat on ice. Barbra couldn't see why; after all, he wasn't having all this stuff done to him! Seeing inside her body on the ultrasounds made Barbra anxious and slightly sick to her stomach, but she felt that any woman would probably want to see them, so she suffered in silence.

Barbra and Cory's studious calculation of the expense of ART was wise. The average cost *per cycle* is $12,400 (according to the

American Society for Reproductive Medicine). Some states require health insurance companies to cover infertility treatment, including ART, but for the majority of Americans these are out-of-pocket costs. (You would need to check with your own insurance company.) Barbra was fortunate to have paid leave to use while adjusting to the side effects. For working women who need to keep working during ART, it is usually possible to manage the hormonal treatments, ultrasounds, and other procedures while working, although you will need a few days off around the time of egg harvesting.

After the eggs are retrieved, they are fertilized in the laboratory using sperm produced by the woman's partner. This is done by masturbation if the man has normal function or by one of the techniques described above (TESA, MESA) if there is a blockage. Alternatively, if the man has no sperm at all (a condition known as azoospermia), donor sperm may be used. The resulting zygotes are incubated for 24 hours then inspected to confirm that fertilization has occurred. By 48 hours, the embryo should have divided into four cells; this is the point at which most clinics transfer the embryo into the woman's uterus. Some clinics wait longer and do the transfer at 5 to 6 days, the blastocyst stage, usually because they plan to do some genetic tests before transferring the embryos. Current practice is to transfer not more than two embryos per cycle, to avoid the possibility that the pregnancy will produce triplets or even greater numbers of babies. Extra embryos may be frozen (cryopreservation) to be used in subsequent cycles.

Preimplantation genetic diagnosis (PGD) is a technique in which a very few cells are taken from a developing embryo before transfer into the uterus and examined to see whether the usual number of chromosomes is present. (PGD is similar to the testing for Down syndrome and other conditions, described in Chapter 10.) PGD can also be used to test for the presence of inheritable (genetic) conditions known to exist in either parent's family. If markers for a serious condition are present, the mother and her partner may decide not to have that embryo transferred. "Healthy" embryos are those most likely to successfully implant and to proceed to grow normally into healthy babies. PGD is an optional procedure. Some people have religious objections to the technique itself and to the selection process it enables. If you have concerns of this sort, you may wish to consult with your religious advisors.

Another technique that may improve, at least marginally, the chances of successful implantation of the embryo is called "assisted hatching." A small opening is made in the outer layer of the embryo, by means of a tiny laser beam; this opening seems to enhance the embryo's attachment to the wall of the uterus. The technique is similar to the gardener's trick of pricking the hard outer shell of some seeds before planting, to encourage germination.

To help support the lining of the uterus during the time when the new embryo is implanting, progesterone is usually given for 10 to 14 days. Progesterone is the hormone produced naturally by the ovaries in the second half of a woman's cycle, so this administration of progesterone mimics what happens in natural conception. Sometimes ultrasound exam shows that the lining of the woman's uterus is not ready for implantation of the embryo and the embryos will be saved until the next cycle.

One side effect of ART can be the hyperstimulation of the ovaries, producing cysts—collections of fluid—which can burst, causing pain, vomiting, and distension of the abdomen. Sometimes these symptoms are so severe that hospital admission is required. This is less of a problem than it used to be, because we now understand better how to "fine-tune" what's happening in the ovaries, monitoring with ultrasound and adjusting the hormone doses. Twin pregnancy is still common, however. When two embryos are transferred into the uterus, usually one does not develop, and a single baby (called a "singleton") results. In about 20 percent of cases, however, both embryos develop. The rate of twins in mothers receiving ART is about twenty times that of the general population. Many couples are delighted to have twins, but, as we will explain in Chapter 19, these pregnancies have more risk than singleton pregnancies and there is a greater possibility of losing both babies.

In the last step of a cycle of ART, the embryo or embryos are introduced into the uterus by means of a tiny cannula (tube) passed through the cervix. Generally this process takes only a few minutes and is no more uncomfortable than having a Pap smear taken.

In women over 35, clinical pregnancy results in about 30 percent of women after a single cycle of ART, and the baby is delivered successfully in 15 to 20 percent of these cases. Success rates decrease, however, with the age of the woman; and in women over 42, only about 2 percent produce live births if the woman's own eggs are used. (We'll say more about donated eggs below.) Studies of ART records show that a successful pregnancy carried to term takes an average of six cycles. Barbra and Cory are among the lucky ones. They achieved a successful pregnancy on Barbra's second cycle of ART. Only one embryo developed, and Barbra delivered a healthy son at 38 weeks. (Statistically, ART is slightly more likely to produce boys than girls.)

There are variations on this basic ART theme. GIFT, or gamete intra-Fallopian transfer, is the transfer of the egg and the sperm separately into the Fallopian tube, with fertilization taking place in the Fallopian tube; this is feasible only if there is no Fallopian tube disease or blockage. ZIFT, zygote intra-Fallopian transfer, is the transfer of the fertilized egg into the Fallopian tube. In both instances, transfer to the Fallopian tubes is technically similar to harvesting the eggs. Again, the woman needs to have healthy, patent Fallopian tubes. GIFT and ZIFT are rarely used now; we mention them because you may have friends who have had these procedures or you may come across them in your reading. Also, as we mentioned, when a cycle of regular IVF is unsuccessful in couples where there is no apparent problem with the man's sperm, it may be decided that in the next cycle ICSI will be used to try to achieve fertilization, because this has been shown to be useful in some cases.

Using Donor Eggs and Sperm

We have touched on the use of donor sperm or eggs. For a woman over age 42, pregnancy is most likely to occur if eggs donated by a younger woman are used. Her chance of conceiving and carrying a baby to term using her own eggs in ART is 2 percent or less; for women aged 40 to 42, it is 14 percent or less. Spontaneous abortion (miscarriage) rates are high (about 40%) in this age group, presumably because of the high incidence of abnormal ova. Experts agree that a woman in this age group has the best chance of a successful term pregnancy if she uses donor eggs. Eggs may be donated by family or friends or obtained from anonymous donors through fertility clinics, where there are usually waiting lists. An egg donor goes through an ovulation stimulation and egg harvesting under anesthetic, so the process is not without risk for her. Use of donor sperm is recommended only if the male parent has no sperm or has abnormal sperm or if there is no male parent. Donor sperm is produced by masturbation within the clinic setting. Obviously, the donor should be screened for sexually transmitted and other communicable diseases; in addition, his own medical history should be known and recorded, as should any relevant family history. Much thought and discussion should precede the decision to use donated sperm or eggs. In some cases, both are used.

ETHICAL AND LEGAL QUESTIONS

Assisted reproductive technology is fraught with difficult ethical issues. We have no perfect answers and there are no comforting one-size-fits-all responses. Some—but by no means all—of the questions that you may need to consider for yourself are:

- If I use donor eggs, will I be the birth mother? the natural mother? What rights has the genetic mother regarding my baby? What claims will my baby have on the genetic mother? How can I ensure that this child when grown does not make babies with his or her half-sibling?
- What are the answers to the same questions if I use donor sperm?
- What happens to the unused embryos? If they are destroyed, is this moral? If they are donated, all the previous questions pertain again. (The issue of preventing future progeny from people born of donated embryos is even more important, because the resultant people are full genetic siblings, not just half-siblings.)

- If I divorce, how does this affect my child legally?
- Will my child be more prone to certain abnormalities? (We really know very little as yet about the long-term effects of being conceived artificially.)

You can probably add many more questions to this list, and more will arise as you explore this treatment. You see how difficult this can become.

The Emotional Toll

Be mindful that a tremendous emotional toll can be exacted by the cycle-to-cycle swings of hopefulness and grief, even if they are eventually followed by triumph. It takes a strong relationship to hold up under these stresses. Besides the natural emotional aspects of all of this, you will also be subject to yo-yo mood swings because of the hormones used in ART. Here are a couple of stories of real people that illustrate what we're talking about.

Sydney was a teacher, in fact she was head of a prestigious private high school. She and Tom had married in their mid-thirties and were busy with their careers until, when Sydney was 41, they realized that they wanted to have a family before it was too late. Their doctor recommended an immediate referral for in vitro fertilization because of Sydney's age. They approached the whole process with complete optimism; they were sure that none of the difficulties the doctor kept talking about would apply to them. Six cycles of IVF later, they were at each other's throats and still were not pregnant. Sydney was ready to try one more cycle, but Tom was very skeptical about the possibility of success. When their arguing accelerated, they terminated the ART and entered counseling to see if they could hold together the shreds of their marriage.

Lisa and her husband, Seth, were a different story. They had married straight out of college and had begun trying to start a family soon thereafter. Lisa was tormented by endometriosis and alternated treatment for that with attempts to conceive. When she was 33, she became pregnant but miscarried almost as soon as she realized she was pregnant. Both Lisa and Seth were devastated. They were too disheartened to try again to conceive for quite some time. When Lisa was 38, they decided to look into IVF and maybe donor eggs, since involvement of her ovaries in the endometriosis seemed to be part of the problem. They knew from what they'd already been through and from their reading that this would not be a walk in the park, so they started couples counseling with a therapist attached to the infertility clinic they had chosen. The support proved helpful, strengthening their relationship. At age 40, Lisa gave birth to a healthy baby boy. Yes, half of his genetic material came from another woman, for they had used donated eggs, but Lisa knew that she was his mother in all the ways that mattered and that she had nurtured him under her heart.

Sometimes things work out as a couple wishes and sometimes they do not; part of approaching pregnancy over 35 is being prepared for either outcome. If you receive cautions about ART from your doctor, do not dismiss them. Your doctor knows you and knows that ART can significantly affect a woman's emotional and physical health, and might also put a considerable strain on your relationship and finances, so she or he will wish you to weigh carefully all the pros and cons before embarking on this way of achieving motherhood.

Elaine is a librarian, aged 43. She was in a new relationship with Mac, had never been pregnant, and began to think that it might not be too late after all. After several months of trying, she was still not pregnant, and her family doctor sent her to talk to the ART people in the nearest city. Elaine had already done some research on the Internet and knew that she might need donor eggs; she has a younger sister who had agreed to provide eggs for her. However, Dr. Robson, a woman with twelve years experience in ART, sat down and had a long and frank discussion with Elaine and Mac. She pointed out that Elaine weighed in excess of 265 pounds and had chronic hypertension requiring two different medications. These factors make the

ART process more hazardous and they are significant impediments to successful pregnancy. The doctor sent them off with instructions to think about it all. Over dinner that night, Mac firmly asserted that he did not want them to do anything that would risk Elaine's health, and thus her happiness and his, especially when there was no guaranteed outcome of a live and healthy baby. The upshot was that they decided to become short-term foster parents, with the idea of proceeding to long-term fostering if this goes well.

There are many different paths to motherhood, and we discuss them in Chapter 9.

POSTMENOPAUSAL PREGNANCY

Many readers will have heard of the Italian woman of 63 who gave birth to a son by means of ART, after the tragic death of the son she had had years earlier. She underwent hormonal stimulation of her uterus, which, after the menopause (by definition, the last normal period of a woman's life) becomes small and inactive, and she used donor eggs.

In theory this treatment is possible at any age. However, most women, their partners, and their doctors would not choose it beyond somewhere between ages 45 and the early fifties. (In Michele's family, the story is told of her mother-in-law, then a sprightly lady in her early eighties, appearing at breakfast to report that she'd dreamt she was pregnant—"at my age! Thank goodness it was just a dream!") All the cautions for women in the over-35 category apply increasingly with every year of age. In addition to looking at all the medical realities, an older woman needs to calculate and honestly confront how old she will be when she is caring for a toddler, a grade schooler, and finally a teenager.

Overview of ART for Older Women

- A woman's age is a very important prognostic factor for the success of ART.
- Women over the age of 40 have fertility rates 50% lower than those of younger women. Even though the effectiveness of IVF and ICSI techniques has improved over the past 15 years, they are still less successful in older women.
- Oocyte quantity and quality decrease with age.
- Cumulative conception, implantation, and live birth rates following IVF decline significantly with age. Success after five cycles of IVF is 54% at age 20, 45% at age 34, 38% at age 35, 29% at age 39, 20% at 40, and 2% at 42.
- The use of donor eggs in women over 35 significantly increases the live birth rate.
- IVF pregnancies are associated with high multiple-birth rates, increased risks of bleeding and high blood pressure in pregnancy, and increased rates of preterm birth, Cesarean section, and slowed in-utero growth.
- Pregnancy rates following ICSI are similar to those for IVF.
- There is an increase in Beckwith-Weidemann syndrome in children born via IVF, but it is still rare. Beckwith-Weidemann syndrome is a recognizable grouping of characteristics, some of which are prenatal and perinatal hypoglycemia (low blood sugar), large tongue that may interfere with feeding, large size, and abdominal wall defects. There is also a significant risk of malignancies of the kidneys or liver in persons with this syndrome.
- There is an increased risk of hypospadias in boy babies born by IVF. In hypospadias, the urethra, the tube lining the penis, opens onto the lower surface of the penis instead of at the tip. The condition is nevertheless uncommon and is treatable.

- *So far, studies do not confirm any increased risk of cancer or impaired intellect in babies born by IVF, nor have any long-term side effects been demonstrated in women who have undergone ART, although studies continue.*
- *There are better outcomes if only two embryos are transferred into the uterus.*
- *Single-fetus pregnancies resulting from IVF have more perinatal morbidity and mortality than single-fetus pregnancies conceived naturally.*
- *Past history of infertility increases the risk of perinatal death.*
- *Previous pregnancy with live birth significantly increases the chance of success with ART.*

Chapter 7

———— ❧ ————

Medical Conditions That May Affect Pregnancy

Numerous medical conditions that occur more frequently in women over 35 may affect the course of a pregnancy, or be affected by pregnancy, or both. In this chapter we will deal in detail with the most common of these, including hypertension (high blood pressure) and diabetes, and mention several others. In the next chapter we will address cancers, which unfortunately are not uncommon in women of reproductive age.

Our advice is intended to complement, not replace, that of your own doctors, who know your particular circumstances. They may say that pregnancy is not a good idea for you because there is a definite risk of damaging your own health (and sometimes, indeed, of dying) or because your medical condition makes successful pregnancy unlikely. We suggest you take such advice seriously. There are other ways of becoming a mother (discussed in Chapter 9).

HYPERTENSION

Hypertension, or high blood pressure, is a common problem in many Western societies. It is estimated to affect 2 percent of all women of childbearing age in the United States, but that figure rises with the age of the women being assessed. Hypertension is defined as a blood pressure that, consistently over at least three separate checks, reads 140/90 or higher; borderline high blood pressure is 135/85 or greater. (The upper figure in a blood pressure reading is called "systolic" and the lower figure "diastolic." The numbers refer to millimeters of mercury in a thermometer-like gauge.) Hypertension may develop for the first time during pregnancy. It is a complication in 6 to 8 percent of all pregnancies in the United States.

Hypertension as it relates to pregnancy is divided into four categories: (1) chronic high blood pressure predating pregnancy, (2) gestational hypertension or uncomplicated high blood pressure developing in the second half of pregnancy (after 20 weeks), (3) chronic high blood pressure complicated by preeclampsia, and (4) preeclampsia appearing without any previous known rise in blood pressure.

Preeclampsia is a serious condition that occurs only in women in the second half of pregnancy and is characterized by high blood pressure, protein in the urine, and swelling of feet, legs, hands, and sometimes the face. Women who have preexisting hypertension have a 25 percent risk of developing preeclampsia in pregnancy, and, because high blood pressure is more common in older mothers, so is preeclampsia. Chapter 18 provides information about preeclampsia, and about eclampsia, a dangerous condition characterized by seizures during pregnancy or labor that fortunately is now very rare in countries with good medical care.

For the woman with preexisting hypertension, careful prenatal planning is advised. Ideally, such a woman will maintain her body mass index (see Appendix C) at 26 or less and will have discussed her plan for pregnancy with her doctor. If she is on a blood pressure–lowering medication, her doctor may change it to a drug that is safer for the developing baby. An old drug, methyldopa, is still frequently the drug of choice for hypertensive pregnant women because of its long safety record. Alpha- and beta-blockers are used as alternative drugs today, but ACE inhibitors are not used in pregnancy because of serious adverse effects on the developing baby's kidneys. These effects happen during the second and third trimesters of pregnancy, so if you are on an ACE inhibitor when you get pregnant, don't be overly alarmed; simply make sure that your doctor switches you to something else well before the second trimester (this means by about 12 weeks of pregnancy). If you have any questions about your particular medication, ask your health care provider. The National High Blood Pressure Education Program's

Working Group states that hypertensive women with no signs of "end organ damage," systolic blood pressure no higher than 179, and diastolic no higher than 109 can be managed safely without drugs during pregnancy. ("End organ damage" means damage to the kidneys, which would be indicated by protein in the urine, or damage to the retina at the back of the eye, which can be checked by your doctor using an ophthalmoscope.) Obviously, any changes in your blood pressure during pregnancy would be cause for reevaluation of the need for medication.

Hope is a successful woman by anyone's criteria. She is managing editor at a large publishing house and has deferred pregnancy in order to pursue her career goals. Since the age of 33, Hope has taken an ACE inhibitor for high blood pressure, which has been prevalent in her family and is not helped by the stresses of her daily life. Now 38, Hope is pregnant and is suddenly aware that her "little high blood pressure" may be a significant complication for her pregnancy. After some initial alarm, Hope came to feel that she could manage pregnancy as well as she had everything else in her life and that all would go well. She was nervous about her doctor's recommendation that she go off all medication and monitor her blood pressure frequently, with the plan to use a different drug if medication seemed necessary. She had read that methyldopa could cause depression, and she certainly had no time for that side effect. Dr. Hassan explained that, because she was at increased risk of preeclampsia, she would be monitored closely for protein in her urine and an early sonogram would be done to confirm her expected date of delivery and as a baseline to monitor the growth of her baby. She also had kidney function tests to detect any hidden abnormality there and had her eyes checked. Fortunately all these tests were normal.

We will tell you more about Hope and the progress of her pregnancy in a later chapter.

Diabetes

Diabetes is an increasingly common problem in developed Western societies. Diabetes is a malfunctioning of the body processes that metabolize carbohydrates, and it occurs when there is a lack, absolute or relative, of the pancreatic hormone insulin. An absolute lack would constitute the failure of the pancreas, an organ that sits behind the stomach and produces insulin. A relative lack is a disproportion between the amount of insulin being produced and the amount needed by the body. In obese people, the demand by the body tissues for insulin exceeds the body's ability to produce it. A factor that complicates things is that sometimes the tissues become insensitive to the action of insulin; enough insulin is being produced, but it isn't having the intended effect. Insulin helps to maintain the glucose or sugar levels in your blood and thus the amount of glucose cells have to use as fuel—glucose is the energy source for body tissues. A lack of insulin or lack of sensitivity to insulin leads to higher than normal blood sugar levels—hyperglycemia. (Insulin has other complex roles in the functioning of our metabolism, but these are beyond the scope of this book. Many good books about diabetes are available in your library and bookstores, and information is available from the American Diabetes Association.)

We will refer to three types of diabetes: Type 1, or juvenile-onset diabetes; Type 2, or adult-onset diabetes; and gestational diabetes, or diabetes that shows up during pregnancy. Any of these can be a problem in pregnancy.

Type 1 diabetes usually occurs in children or young adults and is caused by an absolute inability of the pancreas to produce enough insulin. Because of this, the person is dependent upon insulin injections once or sometimes multiple times during the day. Most people with Type 1 diabetes rapidly learn to test their blood sugars several times daily and to give themselves their insulin injections. They learn to balance their food intake and exercise and insulin requirements. Also, they know that stress, be it physical, such as an infection, or emotional, will affect their blood sugar levels and therefore their need for insulin. Pregnancy is a stressor, both physiologically and emotionally.

Type 2 diabetes is much more common, and unfortunately is increasingly so because of our sedentary lifestyles and our eating habits. We are simply giving our bodies more fuel than is needed and than can be used in a normal manner. Our insulin production cannot keep pace with our calorie intake and our increased body mass. Because in Type 2 diabetes the pancreas is still functioning, although struggling, people with this condition can often control their blood sugars by diet and exercise. A weight loss of as little as 5 to 10 pounds can frequently make a big difference, especially early in the course of the condition. For many diabetics, oral drugs are used, metformin usually being the first drug implemented. Metformin essentially helps the tissues remain sensitive to and able to utilize the insulin produced by the pancreas. There are many other types of oral hypoglycemic drugs (drugs that lower blood sugar levels). Type 2 diabetics often need multiple drug therapy and sometimes insulin as well. This type of diabetes is also adversely affected by stress and may worsen during pregnancy, requiring insulin for women who had not needed it before. At the time of writing, oral hypoglycemic drugs are not being used during pregnancy, although several studies are ongoing to determine the safety and effectiveness of using metformin in pregnant women.

Gestational diabetes (GDM, for gestational diabetes mellitus) is defined as any degree of glucose intolerance that first occurs or is recognized during pregnancy. It happens in women who, for whatever reason, are ordinarily just getting by on the amount of insulin available to their tissues; pregnancy puts enough additional stress on their systems that it overwhelms the delicate balance between available insulin and body demand. Many of the women who develop GDM have a family history of diabetes or may have had GDM in a previous pregnancy. They may be overweight or have previously borne a baby who weighed 10 pounds or more. Some women who develop GDM have had a child that was stillborn for no obvious reason or had difficulty conceiving because of polycystic ovary syndrome. These are all risk factors for gestational diabetes. Many women who develop gestational diabetes will later become

Type 2 diabetics. Approximately 7 percent of *all* pregnancies today are complicated by gestational diabetes. Since we know that gestational diabetes is more common in older mothers, it is of particular concern to the woman over age 35 and her doctor, and screening is done at appropriate points during pregnancies in older women.

All pregnant women should have a fasting glucose test as part of their initial prenatal blood work. If a woman is at high risk, either because she has any of the risk factors mentioned above or because she is a member of an ethnic group at high risk (African Americans, Hispanic Americans, Native Americans, Asian Americans, and Pacific Islanders), she will be scheduled for a 1-hour glucose tolerance test very soon after her first visit. This test involves drinking 50 grams (almost 2 ounces) of a glucose solution and then waiting an hour, at which time a blood sample will be drawn. If her glucose level at one hour measures 130 milligrams per deciliter (mg/dL) or higher, she will then be scheduled for a 3-hour glucose tolerance test.

In a 3-hour glucose tolerance test, a blood sample is drawn when you have not eaten anything—"fasting"—or drunk anything but water for many hours. Then you drink 100 grams of a glucose test drink (flavored orange or cola and sweeter than most women enjoy). Blood samples are then drawn at 1-hour, 2-hour, and 3-hour intervals. Blood sugar levels should not exceed the following values: fasting: 95 mg/dL; 1-hour: 180 mg/dL; 2-hour: 155 mg/dL; 3-hour: 140 mg/dL. If there are two or more elevated values, a diagnosis of GDM is made. Alternatively, two separate fasting values of 126 or more can be considered diagnostic. We now know that fasting elevations of blood glucose in excess of 105 mg/dL can be associated with a risk of intrauterine death in the last 4 to 8 weeks of gestation and that any degree of GDM increases the risk of increased size of the baby, possibly leading to Cesarean delivery, hypoglycemia in the newborn, neonatal jaundice, low blood calcium levels in the baby, and elevated red blood cell counts. These are all good reasons for doctors and patients to be vigilant in screening and aggressive in controlling blood sugars.

Outside the United States, slightly different methods of testing sugar levels may be used. For example, in Australia, 75 grams of glucose are used in the sweet drink, and the most important glucose (sugar) level, apart from the fasting specimen, is the 2-hour level, which should be less than 8 mmol/litre (as you see, glucose levels can be measured by more than one system). However, the overall aim of testing is the same—to detect women who have developed gestational diabetes and to provide them with appropriate treatment to ensure a healthy baby and a healthy mother.

If the initial screen of blood sugar is normal, women at low risk will be screened again between 24 and 28 weeks gestation. You might be screened again earlier if there was glucose in your urine at any prenatal visit. At one time, measuring glucose in the urine was used as a way of testing for diabetes, but we now know that the test is not sensitive enough; sometimes people who do not have diabetes or impaired glucose metabolism will nevertheless have glucose in their urine. Thus, a perfectly healthy pregnant woman may have urinalysis results that are positive for glucose.

A woman who knows she has Type 1 diabetes will, of course, not need to be screened. She will already be in the habit of checking her blood sugar several times daily and taking insulin as needed. Type 1 diabetics are generally well informed about their condition and realistic about its implications. Wendy is an example.

Wendy has been diabetic since her early teen years and has always known that becoming a mother would present more challenges to her than to her friends. She had an unplanned and unsuccessful pregnancy in her mid-twenties and had since put thoughts of being a mother on the back burner. However, she is now 36 years old and in a committed relationship and is feeling an urgency to at least consider pregnancy.

Because she has lived with diabetes for so long and is well educated about it, Wendy knows that pregnancy would pose a risk to her and to the baby. She knows about the much higher risk of fetal abnormalities and of stillbirth, but she has also been reassured by her doctor that these risks can be minimized by meticulous blood sugar control, something she has become good at over the years. After a rebellious period in her midteens, Wendy settled into an acceptance of her illness that has allowed her to take good care of herself. She maintains her weight at around 130 to 135 pounds, which gives her a normal body mass *index of 25. Every day she measures her blood sugar at least twice and regulates her insulin injections according to the need indicated by her blood sugar readings, using a sliding scale that shows how much insulin to use for various blood sugar readings. She is currently well controlled on one shot of insulin each day, but she remembers times when she had to take insulin as often as three times in a day, so she is not complacent about her control.*

Like many diabetics, Wendy is taking a low dose of a blood pressure pill of the class known as ACE inhibitors, even though she is not hypertensive; it is prescribed for its kidney protective effects. This is an important part of long-term diabetic care because of the significant risk of kidney damage from diabetes. Because taking ACE inhibitors is not advised during pregnancy, Wendy will discontinue hers if she becomes pregnant. She has also started taking a prenatal vitamin containing folic acid, to protect the baby from spinal and brain defects, should she conceive.

Wendy understands that the risk of complications is higher in a diabetic mother — even more so if she's older — and that it is necessary for the woman to work in close partnership with her doctor to minimize these very real risks.

Accepting these risks and dealing realistically with them and with diabetes self-care is much harder for women who haven't been living with diabetes most of their lives, as Type 1 diabetics like Wendy have.

Clarissa is 40 years old and pregnant for the fifth time. She has been diabetic since her last child was born. He weighed 10 pounds, 6 ounces, and she had to have a Cesarean section to bear him. Like too many Type 2 diabetics, Clarissa has not taken her diabetes very seriously; she has seen the dietitian several times and knows, in theory, what she should and should not eat, but it is hard to feed a growing family and take care of young children on a tight budget. Clarissa often skips meals and fills up on bread and snacks. Her only exercise is chasing small children, and she feels tired much of the time. She hasn't seen her doctor as regularly as she should; in fact, she goes in only when she has to get a new prescription for metformin.

At her first prenatal visit, Clarissa had the usual tests but was not given a glucose tolerance test, because she was already known to have Type 2 diabetes. She was advised to tighten up her diet, walk for half an hour every day, and use her glucometer: "It is a very good tool to help monitor your blood sugar, but it doesn't work if you never take it out of its case," her doctor reminded her.

Clarissa was sent to see the diabetic educator and the dietitian. The educator again instructed her in the use of a glucometer and told her to test her blood sugar at least twice daily, in the morning and afternoon, until her next appointment in one week. She was taken off metformin, because it is not currently used during pregnancy (a policy that is being reviewed). The dietitian again spent time with her; together they worked out a healthy diet based on foods that were easily accessible to Clarissa and her family. The educator advised Clarissa that during her pregnancy, diet and exercise would probably not be enough to control her blood sugars and that she would probably need sliding scale insulin coverage and more frequent blood sugar monitoring. The implications of a high blood sugar for her baby were explained. Clarissa left the office motivated by the need to keep her baby healthy.

Any woman who has impaired glucose metabolism, regardless of type, *must* do home blood sugar monitoring. Depending on the particular circumstances prevailing in your area, your obstetrician may follow your diabetes in pregnancy or she or you may prefer that you continue to be followed by your family doctor or endocrinologist. Certainly, diabetes in pregnancy makes that pregnancy high-risk, and you should be followed by and deliver in a high-risk obstetrics center where there are also adequate facilities for your baby, who may need special care.

Blood sugar crosses the placenta to the baby, so the mother's blood sugar level directly affects the baby. Insulin, however, is a large molecule that does not cross the placenta, and the baby's body will respond to a high blood sugar from the mother by producing more insulin than normal. One result of this increased insulin is to stimulate growth, which is why babies born to mothers whose blood sugar levels have been higher than optimum are often larger than normal and can require Cesarean section delivery or other operative intervention, such as forceps or vacuum extraction. Also, the newborn may suffer from a drop in blood sugar and need to be given glucose. His serum calcium and/or magnesium may also drop, requiring treatment. Babies of diabetic mothers can be slow in producing surfactant, the substance in the lungs that helps newborns adapt to life as air-breathers. You can see why birth in a center with adequate facilities for high-risk babies is imperative. After all, your baby needs the best start in life.

THYROID DISEASE

Thyroid disease is relatively common in women, and the frequency of hypothyroidism increases with age among women. Thyroid disease can cause infertility, fetal abnormalities, premature labor, and stillbirth. Babies born to mothers with thyroid disease should themselves be checked for thyroid abnormality, which can impair mental development.

*Hypo*thyroidism is a condition in which the person does not have enough thyroid hormone. It is the most common thyroid problem. Any woman feeling abnormally tired, feeling cold, and gaining weight, especially if she has a family history of thyroid disease, should be tested for hypothyroidism. The condition is treated with thyroid hormone medication, in pregnant as well as nonpregnant women. The effectiveness of the treatment is monitored by thyroid function tests, usually measuring two substances: thyroid stimulating hormone (TSH), a pituitary hormone that has an inverse relationship to thyroid hormone; and T_4, or thyroxin, the active form of thyroid hormone, a synthetic version of which is the most common treatment for hypothyroidism.

During pregnancy, a woman taking thyroxin should have a thyroid function test in each trimester, say at 6–8 weeks, 16–20 weeks, and 28–32 weeks, with a recheck 4–6 weeks after any change in the dose of thyroxin. Because of the complex physiologic demands of pregnancy, most women with hypothyroidism will need an upward adjustment of their thyroxin dosage at some point during their pregnancy. Treatment with thyroxin is essentially a replacement therapy, and the medication is safe because it does not cross the placenta into the baby's bloodstream.

Hyperthyroidism, an overabundance of thyroid hormone, affects less than 1 percent of pregnancies and does not seem to affect older women more often than younger women. It is characterized by rapid heart rate, sweating, weight loss, feeling excessively warm, anxiety or nervousness, and diarrhea. It may occur for the first time during pregnancy. Your doctor will test you for hyperthyroidism if your heart rate exceeds 100 beats per minute and/or you are losing weight.

In a pregnant woman, the cause of hyperthyroidism will be diagnosed from the physical exam and from blood tests. In nonpregnant women, nuclear scanning of the thyroid is sometimes done as part of the diagnostic workup, but it must not be done on a pregnant woman, because it could destroy the fetal thyroid gland; the radioactive dye used in this test is taken up by the fetus's thyroid.

In the most common form of hyperthyroidism, Grave's disease, thyroid-stimulating thyroglobulins in the blood will be elevated. Grave's disease, because it is an autoimmune disease, may actually improve during pregnancy, which naturally dampens the mother's immune response.

Hyperthyroidism during pregnancy is usually treated with the drug propylthiouracil, commonly known as PTU. The dose should be the lowest possible that will normalize the thyroid hormone levels and keep thyroid-stimulating thyroglobulins in the normal range. Without treatment, the baby is at risk for spontaneous abortion or premature delivery and the mother is at risk of a phenomenon known as thyroid storm, which can be triggered by any stressor, such as labor, infection, or surgery. Thyroid storm is a life-threatening situation in which the cardiovascular system is tremendously overworked by the circulating thyroid hormone.

The medications given to treat hyperthyroidism do cross the placenta. The baby's thyroid functions should be checked at birth, although they are usually fine.

Rarely, a pregnant woman will not be able to take her hyperthyroidism medication or will require such high doses that it is deemed unsafe for the baby. Then surgical removal of the thyroid may be

recommended. The safest time for this surgery is in the second trimester.

In nonpregnant women, radioactive iodine may be used to destroy the thyroid tissue or beta-blockers may be used to help control
the heart rate. However, beta-blockers should be used only with great
caution during pregnancy, and radioactive iodine absolutely must not
be used by a pregnant woman, because it destroys the baby's thyroid
as well. In follow-up studies, no adverse effects have been noted in
babies whose mothers have taken PTU during pregnancy.

Postpartum autoimmune thyroiditis, or inflammation of the thyroid, can occur in a woman up to one year after delivery. This condition may resolve itself within two years or it may signal the onset
of enduring autoimmune hypothyroidism. If you find that you are
depressed, are more tired than you think you should be (because,
of course, all new mothers are tired), and are having difficulty with
your body thermostat, have a check-up with your doctor.

EPILEPSY

Ninety percent of all pregnancies in women with epilepsy are uneventful. For the other 10 percent, the risks are generally well managed by vigilant and appropriate treatment.

For reasons that are not understood, women whose epilepsy has
been well controlled may experience an increase in seizures during
pregnancy. Because of this, epilepsy treatment must be closely monitored by frequent testing of drug levels in the blood. Optimal control
of epilepsy during pregnancy is vitally important, because seizures can
have serious, even fatal, consequences for both mother and child.

Proper management involves several things:

- Prenatal supplementation with folic acid and vitamin K
- Use of only one antiepileptic drug as therapy, if possible
- Use of the lowest possible dose that will protect against seizure
- Monthly monitoring of blood levels of the chosen medication
- If valproate is used, the dose should be given in three or four
  doses divided over the course of the day.

- If there is any family history of brain or spinal cord defects, neither valproic acid nor carbamazine should be used if there is another drug that is effective.

The doses of folic acid that are recommended to pregnant women with epilepsy—usually 4 mg each day—are higher than the daily 1 mg recommended for other pregnant women. It bears repeating here that all women should begin folic acid supplementation *prior to* conception, whether they have epilepsy or not.

ASTHMA

Asthma affects about 7 percent of all pregnant women. We know of no indication that the incidence is higher in older mothers, but given how common asthma is, we will talk about it here. Studies have shown that asthma worsens during pregnancy in 35 percent of cases, improves in 28 percent, and remains the same in 33 percent. If you had asthma during an earlier pregnancy, you will likely have the same experience you had then. When asthma does get worse, this most commonly happens during the second and third trimesters.

The biggest danger to the baby and the asthmatic mother is undertreatment. Good control ensures normal blood oxygen levels for both the mother and the baby, and the benefits of good blood oxygen levels outweigh any risk from asthma medications.

If you know that your asthma responds to specific triggers, you probably have established how much exposure to your triggers you allow yourself. Pregnancy is a time to increase your avoidance of these triggers.

For Ingrid, eggs are a potent asthma trigger. Before pregnancy, she would weigh her desire for the occasional omelet against the likely sequelae, occasionally indulging and then taking an extra puff from her inhaler. During her pregnancy, however, she was very careful, avoiding dishes in which eggs were an ingredient, knowing that by aggravating her asthma she would be risking not just herself but also her baby.

Appropriate treatment of asthma takes a stepwise approach. The idea is to use as little medication as possible, and the goal is to maintain good control of the disease, to prevent acute episodes rather than have to treat them. The generally accepted treatment for mild, intermittent asthma is an inhaled drug, such as albuterol, used as needed. This would be the approach to, for instance, exercise-induced asthma. Albuterol is considered safe to use during pregnancy, whereas undertreatment or nontreatment of asthma is known to pose a risk.

The next treatment step, added if asthma symptoms are noted more frequently, is a drug like cromolyn or nedocromil, mast cell stabilizers. These drugs are preventive and have shown no adverse effects on the fetus.

If an asthmatic is still having difficulty and her "daily peak flow" measurements are below her desired range, an inhaled corticosteroid is added. The one most commonly used for pregnant women is beclomethasone, because we have the best data about fetal safety for this inhaled steroid.

If asthma attacks continue or peak flow readings are suboptimal, either theophylline or an oral steroid may be added. Theophylline was used much more commonly in the past than it is now. It has the disadvantages of stomach side effects and the need to monitor the blood levels carefully. Also, it interacts negatively with many other medications (not that a pregnant woman should be on a lot of medications) and should not be used during delivery. Oral steroids, when employed, should be tapered as soon as possible to as low a dose as controls the asthmatic symptoms. Often an every-other-day regimen is used. But, again the risks from undertreatment are greater than any posed by the drug.

The stepwise progression of treatment described here is standard in the treatment of asthma in pregnancy. These drugs are also safe to use during breastfeeding.

If an asthmatic mother requires surgical delivery, general anesthesia is avoided. Many obstetricians will choose to utilize an epidural early in labor, to avoid maternal stress and to have adequate analgesia in place if surgical delivery becomes necessary. This is especially important with the older mother, for whom operative delivery is more common.

PREVIOUS THROMBOEMBOLISM

In the chapter about Cesarean section we will discuss deep vein thrombosis (DVT) as a possible side effect of that surgery. In fact, however, DVT is a risk for any pregnant woman, because in pregnancy, there are physiologic changes that enhance the blood clotting mechanisms of the blood, preparing the body for the separation of the placenta and the minor tearing that accompanies most normal deliveries. These changes set the stage for one of the significant causes of maternal mortality—pulmonary embolism. (A thrombus or thrombosis is a blood clot forming within a vein, usually a vein of the legs or pelvis. An embolus is a thrombus that breaks free of its attachment to the blood vessel wall and travels in the bloodstream to a major organ, such as the brain, lungs, or heart, causing serious illness or even death.) Depending upon your source, the figures for occurrence of pulmonary embolus during pregnancy vary from 1 to 7 per every 100,000 births. Besides the normal changes in the blood clotting mechanisms during pregnancy, the pressure of the baby can trigger clotting in the mother's pelvic veins, which transport blood from the legs and pelvis to the heart and the lungs. This is further complicated by the effects of some of the hormones produced by the body during pregnancy, notably progesterone.

Here are the risk factors for deep vein thrombosis and pulmonary embolism:

- Personal history of clotting or presence of antibodies that predispose to clotting. If you have ever had a clot in a leg vein, for example while you were on birth control pills, you are in this category.
- Family history of a clotting disorder or antibodies
- Trauma, especially a fractured or crushed leg (Ski carefully!)
- Being over age 35
- Smoking

- Anemia
- Sickle cell disease
- Surgical delivery

Sometimes, a woman at high risk of clotting problems in her pregnancy will be put on a low dose of injected heparin, a blood thinner. If a woman taking any blood thinner needs anesthesia during delivery, a spinal or epidural anesthetic will have to be avoided because of the risk of bleeding around the spinal cord and resultant damage to the spinal nerves.

At the age of 36, Irene began thinking of having a child. She had experienced two miscarriages in her twenties but didn't worry much about them because she hadn't wanted to be pregnant at the time. During a discussion with her family physician about planning a pregnancy, she mentioned the miscarriages. Her doctor investigated and found that Irene had anticardiolipin antibodies, an indicator of a tendency to develop blood clots. Once her pregnancy was diagnosed, she was started on aspirin (which is safe to use in early pregnancy). At 12 weeks, after an ultrasound scan had shown that everything about the pregnancy looked normal, she began to receive injections of heparin, a drug that helps prevent clotting. Irene's son was born a bit early, because his growth slowed after 30 weeks (a recognized problem in this condition), but he was safely delivered by C-section at 35 weeks under general anesthesia.

CORONARY ARTERY DISEASE

Fortunately, it is rare for a woman of child-bearing age—by definition, premenopausal—to have arteriosclerotic heart disease, but it is possible and, naturally, it is more common among older pregnant women. Any woman who has had a documented heart attack or has had to have bypass surgery should be advised against becoming pregnant. These women should consider other ways of becoming a mother—adoption, surrogacy, fostering (see Chapter 9).

During pregnancy the mother's blood volume is greatly increased, to keep up with the need to supply oxygen and nutrients to the fetus as well as to her own body. This greater blood volume increases the work of the heart from very early in the pregnancy and may make a woman with ischemic heart disease more susceptible to further heart damage.

Rarely, a woman not known to have preexisting heart disease will have a heart attack during pregnancy. Sadly, a heart attack during pregnancy often results in death. Because of this danger, treatment must be aimed at saving the life of the mother, no matter what the stage of gestation.

INFLAMMATORY BOWEL DISEASE

Inflammatory bowel disease (not the same as the less-serious condition irritable bowel syndrome) refers to chronic inflammatory diseases of the intestines, including ulcerative colitis and Crohn's disease. Other terms you may hear are regional enteritis, ileocolitis, and ileitis; these terms generally refer to Crohn's disease. These diseases most often begin when people are in their twenties or thirties. These are illnesses of industrialized nations; they are also more common in whites than in people of color, and most common of all in people of Ashkenazi Jewish heritage. We don't know why.

Inflammatory bowel disease, be it ulcerative colitis or Crohn's disease, is characterized by a waxing and waning of disease symptoms, and the impact on a pregnancy depends on whether the disease is active at the time of conception. If not, the outlook for the pregnancy is very good. If the disease is active, there is some increase in adverse outcomes. The tendency of the disease to remain inactive during the pregnancy if it is inactive at the time of conception may be due to the natural rise in the mother's cortisone-like hormones; the hormones may have a therapeutic effect. In women with ulcerative colitis that is active at the time of conception, the tendency is for the disease to worsen during the pregnancy. Among women with active Crohn's disease at the time of conception, the disease activity remains fairly stable in 60 percent of cases; of the rest, about half improve and half get worse.

Overall, fertility and rates of preterm birth, stillbirth, and developmental defects are about the same as in the general population. This is good news. It is also good that sulfasalazine and steroids, commonly used in treatment of inflammatory bowel disease, are safe to use in pregnancy. Sulfasalazine does interfere with the absorption of folic acid, so women who are taking sulfasalazine should take 1 mg of folic acid twice daily.

Rheumatoid Arthritis

Rheumatoid arthritis is not uncommon among women in their reproductive years. It has traditionally been thought that the symptoms of rheumatoid arthritis improve during pregnancy for most women, and studies have confirmed this; however, in about one-third of affected women, disease symptoms will remain active or may even worsen during their pregnancy. The improvement caused by the pregnancy is unfortunately for the duration of the pregnancy only, and most women relapse after the baby is born. Obviously this sequence of events is very difficult for the mother, who is well advised to have a good support system in place, including help with the care of the baby and her home.

For pregnant women with rheumatoid arthritis, planning is even more important than usual. Many of the drugs used to treat this illness are not safe for a developing fetus, and some do not clear the body quickly. You may need to discontinue them several months *before* becoming pregnant. Of concern are methotrexate, cyclosporine, cyclophosphamide, leflunomide, azathioprine, and gold injections. Ask your doctor about your specific medications well in advance of becoming pregnant. During pregnancy, the preferred drugs to modify the course of the disease are sulfasalazine and hydroxychloroquine. Fish oil supplements can be continued and calcium supplementation is important.

Studies indicate that women with rheumatoid arthritis as compared with other women are no less fertile and have no increased frequency of adverse events during pregnancy or abnormalities, morbidity, or mortality in their babies. They may take longer to

conceive, but this could be due to many factors, among them decreased sex drive because of fatigue or pain, the time required to
wean from drugs, and impaired communication between the pituitary gland and the ovaries. A woman with rheumatoid arthritis is
no more likely to have a surgical birth than any other woman. She
will, of course, have some physical challenges after the birth that
most mothers without this disease will not.

Lupus

The picture is somewhat less rosy for the woman with lupus, which,
like rheumatoid arthritis, is an autoimmune disease common in
women of reproductive age. Half of all women with lupus have successful pregnancies, coming uneventfully to delivery; but 25 percent will deliver prematurely, and fetal loss occurs in the remaining
25 percent. Therefore, if you have lupus and are pregnant, even
if everything seems to be going normally, your pregnancy should
be considered a high-risk pregnancy and you should be followed
by a clinic capable of dealing with the possible consequences. You
should not even think about a home birth or the use of a lay midwife. Your birth should take place in a hospital that has a premature
intensive care nursery or, if it is in a rural area, access to such a unit
on an urgent basis; there are regional centers for the care of high-
risk newborns. Inform yourself about all types of delivery, including
surgical delivery. You are not a good candidate for a water birth or
"all natural" childbirth, because it is not uncommon for complications to occur during delivery, requiring quick intervention.

During your pregnancy, you are unlikely to have a serious flare
of your lupus, and 10 to 15 percent of women will actually improve
temporarily. If you do have a flare, it will most likely be during the
first two trimesters or soon after delivery. If you've been in remission, you are likely to remain so. If possible, time pregnancy during
a remission, or at least, when you are feeling as well as possible. If
you need treatment during your pregnancy, prednisone and pred-
nisolone are safe to use. Other steroids, for instance dexamethasone
and betamethasone, cross the placenta, but they might be used if

there are signs that your baby will be premature, because these ste-roids would help to mature the baby's lungs as well as treat your symptoms. Of the other drugs used, cyclophosphamide is definitely to be avoided. Hydroxycholoroquine may be used, as may aspirin.

There is evidence that women with lupus are more prone to preeclampsia (20% increase) and to the antibodies that can cause blood clots (antiphospholipid antibodies). Because these antibod-ies can cause clotting in the placenta, they are one of the causes of miscarriage. Again, these are good reasons to have only the most expert care.

Neonatal lupus occurs in about 3 percent of babies born of moth-ers with lupus. The baby will have a transient rash, transiently low platelets in the blood (platelets are important for blood clotting), and a particular heart problem, which is treatable but permanent. The heart problem is a conduction block and is diagnosable with an EKG. Neonatal lupus is rare.

Breastfeeding may be unadvisable if you are taking medications that are passed into the breast milk. Ask your doctor for advice in your own case. If your baby was premature and is unable to nurse, and if your doctor says your breast milk is safe, you can pump and freeze milk to give once your baby is able to nurse. Contact the LaLeche League or your local lactation specialist for helpful infor-mation.

Another point for the older mother with lupus to consider is making arrangements for child care during disabling flare-ups of the illness. Realistic care planning prior to conception, or at least before the birth, will decrease the stress of a flare-up after the baby is born. Remember that you can love your child and be his mother even if someone else ties his shoes.

Chapter 8

——— ❧ ———

Pregnancy following Cancer and Precancer

It is not common for a woman under 50 to have cancer, but it is not rare, either, and the frequency of cancer is increasing. Breast cancer and cervical cancer and precancer are the most common types. In the United States, there are approximately 3,500 cancer-complicated pregnancies each year.

Most women who have had cancer have an acutely heightened sense of their own mortality and fear that they may not live to see their child grown. For a woman whose overall prognosis is good, the increased risk of early death is not tremendous. However, each cancer survivor should visit this issue and come to peace with it. If you wish to get pregnant, consider these questions. Will your child have a support system that can sustain him if you should die? Are you in a stable relationship and will your partner be able to parent your child on his or her own? Many children lose their parents to illness, accident, or warfare; how the child fares depends on her or his support network. Michele's sister Maureen died of cancer at age 31, leaving a daughter age 6 and a son age 3. Maureen had time to plan, and she left her children in the care of another sister, with whom they had spent much time during Maureen's illness.

Every woman's story is unique, but cancer almost never shows up at an expected and convenient moment.

Judy married young, and her son Tom was born when she was 24. Her life was good until she and her husband divorced when she was 30, after she found him with her best friend. Single parenting was difficult, but she managed. When Judy was 35, life took an unexpected turn for for the good: she met Rob, an accounts executive in the insurance company where she worked. Rob was a widower in his late forties with two grown sons. After a cautious two-year courtship, Judy and Rob married. On their honeymoon, Rob found a little lump in Judy's breast. Judy was nonchalant about it, telling him, "Oh, that's just a little passing bump; it'll go away with my period, I'm sure. I'm too young to have any real problem." Rob, however, insisted that she see her doctor as soon as they returned home.

The following week, Judy had a biopsy, and cancerous cells were found. She then had a lumpectomy. Her lymph nodes were negative for spread of the cancer; she was given the option of follow-up radiation but decided against it.

Three years later, Rob lost one of his sons in a tragic skiing accident. Judy was as devastated as Rob, and after the initial period of shock, she suggested to Rob that they look into the possibility of having a child of their own, knowing that age and the history of cancer were complications that might make it impossible.

Judy's oncologist and her obstetrician-gynecologist pointed out that Judy had been cancer free for three years and that her cycles had continued, uninterrupted, so there was no strong reason for her not to try to become pregnant. Judy was worried that the high hormone levels that occur during pregnancy might fan a recurrence of the cancer, but her oncologist said that the probability of that was low in her case. Judy's own prognosis was good, based on her tumor type, and the available studies showed that women with similar histories had not been adversely affected by pregnancy. Of course, he qualified, women with poor prognoses had probably avoided pregnancy and this fact would not be reflected in these studies.

Judy and Rob stopped using contraception and set out to get pregnant.

We cannot advise you about your own particular risk; like Judy you need to consult with trusted professionals who know you and your situation in detail.

If Judy had had chemotherapy or radiation that had stopped her menstrual cycles and caused the changes of early menopause, her situation would have been different. If she had been taking tamoxifen, a drug which opposes the effects of estrogen, she would have needed to discontinue it prior to trying to conceive.

Judy conceived after three months of trying and was blessed with an uneventful pregnancy and delivery. She and Rob are now parents of a healthy daughter, Erin, who fills their days with joy. Judy is so thankful that she made the decision to become pregnant. She has also had no difficulty breastfeeding Erin, although her affected breast does seem to give less milk. The one dimming of her joy is that she will one day have to tell Erin that she herself is at greater risk of getting breast cancer.

If a woman is diagnosed with breast cancer during pregnancy, treatment of the cancer has to take precedence, and failure of the pregnancy may end up being a sad outcome of the treatment. Breast surgery during pregnancy is usually safe, and chemotherapy can usually be given with little risk to the fetus in the second and third trimesters. Methotrexate and tamoxifen would not be used. Radiation is to be avoided; other means of imaging than x-rays would be used to check for spread of the cancer.

When a woman has ovarian cancer, the ovaries are usually removed and chemotherapy and/or radiation is given. For these women, alternate means of motherhood are still viable options, including having some of her eggs removed and frozen before surgery. The recent (2004) birth of a healthy baby to a Belgian woman who had her eggs harvested and frozen prior to her treatment for ovarian cancer raises the hope that this technology will make "natural" motherhood feasible for more women in similar circumstances in the future.

Obviously, if the uterus has been removed, a pregnancy cannot be carried. Because of this, a woman who has had a hysterectomy for any type of pelvic cancer—or any other reason—cannot become pregnant. Fortunately, pelvic cancers are relatively rare in women of reproductive age.

Precancerous conditions, in particular precancerous changes in the cervix, are quite common. These are mostly detected as a result of Pap smear screening. Pap smears detect precancerous changes in the cells of the cervix and allow treatment of these lesions before they progress to actual cancer. As a result of Pap smear screening, death rates from cervical cancer in American women have plummeted in the past forty years.

Abnormalities on Pap smears are relatively common and often prompt a colposcopic exam and biopsy of the areas that look abnormal. The colposcope is an instrument by which the doctor can see the cells on the cervix and vagina under magnification. If these exams indicate any significant abnormalities or precancerous changes, treatment is necessary. Treatment may consist of: (1) laser or diathermy, which destroy the abnormal tissue with either a concentrated beam of light energy or heat; (2) LEEP or LLETZ procedures, which use a hot wire to remove the abnormal tissue in a single piece; or (3) cone biopsy, which consists of surgically removing a cone-shaped portion from the lower cervix and then suturing the raw edges of the cervix.

These treatment procedures are very effective at removing tissue that shows precancerous change, but occasionally the change may recur, necessitating repetition of the procedure. These treatments are now common in women aged 25 to 35, so many women hoping to conceive after 35 will have had such treatments and wonder how they will affect their chances of successful pregnancy.

A single laser, diathermy, LEEP, or LLETZ procedure has not been shown to have any deleterious effect on the functioning of the cervix in getting pregnant or maintaining the pregnancy (the cervix needs to stay closed while the baby is growing in the uterus and then respond to the signals to dilate to allow delivery of the baby). In a single instance of one of these procedures, a very small amount of tissue is involved and the competency of the cervix is not compromised.

However, a cone biopsy or multiple procedures may compromise the function of the cervix. This is because more tissue is taken and the cervix may be shortened, making it looser and less effective at staying closed, a condition, called "cervical incompetence," which makes premature labor or miscarriage more likely. Alternatively, following a cone biopsy the cervix may be tighter or closed by scar tissue in a condition called "cervical stenosis," making it difficult for sperm to get through to fertilize the egg. If pregnancy does oc-cur, such scarring of the cervix may keep the cervix from dilating properly during labor, requiring a Cesarean section.

If you have had any of these procedures done and are pregnant, it is important that you talk to your doctor about the possibility of these complications. She or he can watch you more closely for signs of cervical incompetence. Some doctors may want to put in a "purse string" type of suture; although this practice is common, there is little research evidence that it actually improves cervical competence. If there is much scarring of your cervix, your doctor may recommend a planned C-section for delivery.

You may have had one of these treatments and be concerned that you will develop a higher-grade cervical lesion while you are pregnant. This is extremely unlikely if you have had follow-up Pap smears and/or colposcopy, if indicated. Cervical lesions are slow growing, and in 90 to 95 percent of cases are completely removed by the treatments discussed above. Unless you have just had a Pap smear, that test will be part of your initial prenatal visit. It is smart to have regular Paps, but if you've overlooked this, having one prior to conceiving will give you time to treat anything that might be found before getting pregnant.

The other cancers that most frequently complicate pregnancy are melanoma, cancer of the thyroid, leukemia, lymphoma, and colorectal cancer. They are all much less common than breast and cervical cancer, so we will treat them as a group. In general, if these cancers are diagnosed during pregnancy, they must be treated; the cost to the mother of delaying treatment is too great. Radiation is to be avoided, if possible. Many chemotherapeutic drugs can be used fairly safely; having an experienced team of obstetricians and oncologists will minimize the risks to the fetus. It is beyond the scope of this book to discuss the impact of each of these cancers on a pregnancy. A good team of specialists will be able to assess your situation and minister to your particular needs.

Happily, according to studies, the children of cancer survivors do not seem to be at increased risk for birth defects or genetic dis-orders. Although cancer treatment does not increase any of these risks, children should receive counseling in early adult life about any possible inherited disorders. In some cases, genetic counseling and perhaps preventive surveillance should begin earlier than usual. Familial polyposis, in which colon cancer may develop at a very early age, is a prime example.

Clearly, if this chapter applies to you, your pregnancy will benefit from a team approach, using the skills of your oncologist, your obstetrician, and your pediatrician. Encourage them to discuss your case with you and with each other, and know that all involved want you to have a good outcome.

Chapter 9

————— ∾ —————

Other Roads to Motherhood

Growing a baby inside your own uterus is not the only way to become a mother. Women adopt children, become stepmothers, foster parent other people's children, and arrange for a surrogate to bear a child for them. These are alternative roads to motherhood, but the destination is the same.

STEPMOTHERHOOD

When a woman marries someone who has children, she becomes those children's stepmother. Young children are usually prepared to love anyone who is open to loving them; older children may be more reluctant, because their loyalties are formed and they don't always have the maturity to know that the heart is an incredibly elastic organ, accommodating enough love for many people.

We must tell you about our friend Ros, a doctor who, when she was 40, met and married Dennis. Dennis had four children with his first wife, who, sadly, had died from breast cancer when their youngest child was an infant. Dennis married a second wife, a lovely woman with three young children. Tragically, this woman also died, from a cerebral hemorrhage within two years of their marriage. So, when Ros married Dennis, she became stepmother to a brood of seven—a task she has managed with extraordinary skill and humor ever since.

Ros made a very important point to us: stepmothers must realize that children need to love and remain loyal to their birth mother, even if she has died. You can be a wonderful bonus in their lives—a second mother that they love equally but differently from their first mother—but only if you acknowledge their need to preserve that bond. If their birth mother is living, you will need to carefully balance your role with their other mother's. The presence of both of you can enrich the children's lives. If their mother has died, they need to preserve her memory; and if they were very young when she died, stories of her will be important to them. Preserving your stepchildren's bond with their birth mother in no way detracts from your relationship with them and will probably strengthen it.

ADOPTION

Adoption is a wonderful way to become a mother. It satisfies powerful needs of at least two people: your need to be a parent and the child's need to have a parent. Many children in this world have been deprived of loving parents by illness, war, famine, abandonment, or any of countless other tragedies. The children are innocent and need love and nurturing to flourish and become the best person they can be.

Your adoptive child is your own child as truly as any child you might have borne in your body. Ask Rena.

Rena gave birth to three daughters while she was still in her twenties, and she was happy with her family. When she was 37, she heard of a baby boy who had been abandoned by his drug-addicted birth mother. Rena talked with her husband all night for several nights, and finally they decided to take this baby into their family. Zach is now 17 years old. Rena and her husband have shed many tears over his difficulties, because he was born with fetal alcohol syndrome and crack addiction, but they have never regretted their decision to adopt him. As Rena has often observed, babies don't come with guarantees, no matter how they come to you. Zach is as much their child as their daughters are, and they don't think of him as adopted.

Many couples who adopt already have one or more children. For others, it is a constructive, compassionate response to quite different circumstances.

Everything in Catherine's life seemed to be on schedule: her career was exactly where she'd planned at this point and she and Robert had enjoyed lots of exciting trips and had bought a house. Having a baby was the next scheduled event. After a mostly uneventful pregnancy, Catherine developed eclampsia during labor and the baby died. This trauma plunged her into a deep depression, and she was in therapy for the next two years. Robert was also very sad, but he was able to support her emotionally until she was better. On their 15th wedding anniversary, when Catherine was 37, Robert suggested that they look into adoption: "I'm not a macho type who thinks my child has to have my own genes to carry on my name. I just want a child to love and raise." Adoption was not a quick process, but two years after they applied, their beautiful little daughter, Cileia, who was 18 months old, arrived from Brazil to join their family.

If you adopt a child from another country or culture or a child of a race different from your own, there are a few additional factors to consider. Some people question whether these children can be raised in a culturally appropriate manner. We are certain that having a loving family will offset any cultural disjuncture. Many children who are adopted from a foreign country later visit their birth country, even seeking out their birth mother, and are encouraged and sometimes financially assisted in this quest by their adoptive parents. Some agencies that handle many adoptions of children from other countries run programs that teach children the customs and even the language of their birth country, or can refer you to such a program.

In an earlier chapter we mentioned Louise and Ted, who alternated being the primary caregiver for their son, Owen, in his early years.

Ted and Louise had researched their options carefully and eventually chose private adoption. They contacted a lawyer, who placed ads for them in several states. A pregnant woman contacted them by a toll-free telephone number that they had dedicated to this purpose. They first interviewed the woman on the telephone and then talked with her in person at a meeting set up by the lawyer. The young woman met their criteria, and she agreed that they could adopt her child. Through-

out the pregnancy, Ted and Louise maintained personal contact, by telephone, with the birth mother. According to their contractual arrangement with her, they paid the expenses of her pregnancy. The young woman was living at home with her parents, and when she went into labor, her mother called Ted and Louise and they drove to the hospital for the birth. Everything went as planned and they were able to meet Owen as he took his first breath.

It is not our intention to discuss the details of adoption—practical, ethical, and otherwise—in this book. Be mindful that there are as many variables to consider in adopting as there are in bearing a child and that each family's experience is unique. There are rules for each type of adoption, and each agency or facilitator will have its own policies. These policies will influence your experience, as will the circumstances of the child whom you choose to bring into your home. Interview several agencies, and choose a legitimate agency or facilitator that clearly has the welfare of the child as the highest priority. You and your spouse or partner need to be honest with yourselves about your personal requirements: Jane could not think of taking a child older than an infant; for Marcie, the child could be up to 5 years old, but she knew she wanted a child of her own race; Edie wanted any child under 5 years old and was delighted by her part-Caribbean, part-Mexican daughter.

A very special kind of adoption happens in some ethnic and cultural groups, in which children are viewed as belonging to the community or the extended family instead of to the nuclear family only. These may not be formal adoptions but an extension of the caretaking arrangement, in which a child may say, "My mommy is Betty, but I live with my mommy who's my grannie and I visit my mommy on the weekend. I have two mommies." Or the other mother may be an aunt or an older sister or some other relative. Many children have lived happily and healthily in these arrangements. Sometimes, in these cultures, women who can't bear children are "given" a child to raise by a relative who is blessed with many. Both mothers love these children. If you are a part of one of these traditions, perhaps this kind of motherhood will be available to you.

Surrogacy

The idea of surrogate pregnancy is credited to a lawyer named Noel Keane who thought that women could help each other achieve their dreams of motherhood. However, in cultures like those just mentioned, surrogacy has been quietly practiced for a long time. One sister may have been barren through many years of marriage, so the other sister lies with her sister's partner with the specific purpose of conceiving a child that will then belong to the first sister and her partner, who will be the biological father. In the Bible, did not Hagar bear a child by Abram for Sarah, her mistress?

Surrogacy basically involves a woman bearing a child for another woman. If you were to choose this path, there are several ways it might be accomplished:

1. The surrogate can be artificially inseminated with your partner's sperm.

2. Your egg and your partner's (or a donor's) sperm can meet in a test tube and the resulting embryo can be implanted in the host mother's uterus.

3. A donor egg and your partner's (or a donor's) sperm can be used to make the embryo that is implanted in the host mother.

Any of these may be "open" (that is, the parties know each others' identities) or "closed" transactions, with an intermediary acting on your behalf in closed transactions.

Trudy, whose youngest child was in high school, found out that close family friends were having fertility problems. Although Trudy was herself 35 years old, she considered herself a "Mother Earth" type—she had never had trouble getting pregnant or any problems during her pregnancies and deliveries—so she offered to be a surrogate for her friends. Trudy liked being pregnant and welcomed the chance to experience it once more without embarking on the task of raising another child. She carried the baby, conceived by in vitro fertilization using donor eggs and the sperm of the male partner, in her uterus. She went into labor at 39 weeks and delivered a healthy baby girl.

Surrogacy raises many issues beyond the scope of this book, including the child's ultimate right to know his or her genetic parentage for reasons of future reproductive or medical concerns. Any surrogacy arrangement should include a legal contract drawn up by a lawyer, and the parental rights of the surrogate must be specifically addressed in the contract. This is true even if the surrogate is a friend or family member. As the parent who will raise the child, you will be expected to bear all of the medical costs of the pregnancy and delivery and usually pay a fee to the surrogate. Before committing yourself, find out if the contract that you are anticipating will be legally binding in your state and the state where the surrogate resides, if different.

Carefully consider and then write down the criteria that determine a good surrogate for you. Of course, she needs to be healthy. Beyond that, do you require a high IQ, athletic prowess? Are you looking for particular physical characteristics? Do you want to meet the surrogate or remain anonymous? How much can you afford to pay her? Do you have any emotional reservations about this way of becoming a mother? At the back of the book, in the resources section, you will find helpful addresses and Web sites listed.

FOSTER PARENTING

Being a foster mother is a very special type of parenting. It entails the probable departure from your life of a child whom you've grown to love. At the start of the new millennium, more than half a million children were in foster care; their average stay in any one home was about two and a half years. Foster children range in age from infancy to teenage. A foster mother is appointed by an agency of government, usually the state, to be the temporary guardian and caretaker for the child. If you are the foster mother, you are expected to do for the child all that a biological mother would do. Sadly, not all foster parents love or even like their foster children, and this compounds the emotional damage that these children suffer. A loving foster mother has to have great emotional elasticity, because her heart is stretched to breaking many times, as the children are returned to parents or adopted. Sometimes a foster parent will be able to adopt the child she cares for, but it is unrealistic to enter the system of foster care with this expectation.

A foster mother can be of any age and can be single or married; she is required to have room in her home for a foster child but is not required to own her home. Although she will receive a stipend in compensation for the care of the child, she and her family are required to have another source of income. For the woman who has a strong nurturing instinct and an ability to let go when the child is returned to his parents—which is, after all, the stated goal of the foster care system—being a foster mother can be very rewarding.

Ellen had two biological children and had fostered children all through the years of her marriage. When her husband died at age 52, Ellen had two foster children at home. One, John, had been with her since he was 9 and was then 17. Years later, John still lives with Ellen. She is the only real mother he has ever known, and now he looks after her. She still receives Christmas cards and phone calls from other children whom she fostered. "For me," says Ellen, "this is the reward."

Any of these roads to motherhood can be exactly right for the right person. Assess the advantages and disadvantages carefully before choosing for yourself. For each option, sources of helpful information are available, some of which are listed in the Resources section of this book. We wish you all good fortune with your choice.

Part Three

❧

BEING PREGNANT

_____

Chapter 10

———— ∾ ————

Screening for Chromosomal Abnormalities

Being pregnant and expecting a baby are wonderful. At the same time, most couples are apprehensive to a greater or lesser degree. No one can guarantee a 100 percent perfect baby. Life is not like that. Things can go wrong in the most apparently normal and uneventful pregnancies and labors. Concern on the part of parents about the outcome of pregnancy is understandable regardless of the woman's age.

Two of the main concerns of the older pregnant woman are the possibility that her baby may not be healthy and the possibility of miscarriage. These are normal concerns, and when a mother is older, there *are* increased chances of both miscarriage and problems with the baby's health. We hasten to say that most babies are healthy and most mothers deliver successfully. Still, to prepare you in case something does go wrong, and so you can feel more confident, we will go over some of the things that can go wrong, before we describe a normal pregnancy, labor, and birth.

As we will discuss in detail later, certain medical conditions that are more common in older mothers may be associated with abnormalities in the fetus if they are not recognized and well managed. A good example is diabetes that is not well controlled. Also, some techniques of assisted reproduction, which may be needed by a woman over 35 in order to achieve pregnancy, are associated with a small increase in the number of abnormalities that occur. Clinics providing assisted reproduction often offer testing for these conditions at an early stage once pregnancy has been confirmed.

Your doctors are your best allies in working toward a healthy

pregnancy and baby. They are committed to a good outcome—
mainly in the interests of their patients but also for the sake of their
professional reputations and, to be perfectly frank, for legal reasons,
as well. A happy, healthy baby is the most highly desired outcome
by all involved.

Ana is a very healthy woman, now aged 38, who had delayed conception because she wanted first to be successful in her career in advertising. Now, she is. Her husband, Kenyon, is superintendent of
schools for a nearby district and is as committed to their 15-year marriage as she is. They are financially secure and had planned to have
a child "someday." A little over a year ago, Ana decided that "someday" had arrived. Kenyon was a little more reticent, but he warmed
to the idea. In fact, he acted like a honeymooner, sending beautiful
flowers to Ana at her office every week and picking up little delicacies
to bring home.

It took about six months of attempting conception, while Ana's
anxiety about her fertility rose, but finally she saw the double blue
lines on the home pregnancy test. Overnight, all of Kenyon's ambiva-
lence disappeared. One would think he had invented fatherhood, or, at
least, expectant fatherhood. Although they made a pact to wait until
after the first trimester to tell family and friends—just in case—each
of them confided in several other people, whom they swore to secrecy.
By the time the big announcement was made at a family party, everyone already knew.

As the pregnancy proceeded, Ana became more and more anxious.
She had a sense of having no control over her body and its little resi-
dent. She now liked to eat things that had previously been distasteful
to her; she could not control her waking and sleeping patterns; coffee,
which she loved, made her violently ill—even the smell of it. While
Kenyon became more and more euphoric, Ana worried more. Maybe
all these things meant that there was something terribly wrong with
the baby? Being the "take charge" woman that she is, she borrowed
from the library a book about birth defects and spent a lot of time doing research on the Internet. Soon she began to have true nightmares.
Not only did she accept every test her doctor offered, but she began
to wonder if there were more things she could do to find out what was

going on. Meanwhile, the baby just quietly grew, and all the tests were normal. It was a great relief to all involved when she went into labor and had an uneventful birth of a very healthy baby boy.

Many tests can be done during pregnancy to identify problems with the fetus as early as possible. If they are discovered, some couples will decide to terminate the pregnancy, while other couples will want to obtain information so they can plan for possible consequences. And sometimes, therapeutic intervention is an option. Regardless, the sooner potential problems are discovered, the better. This book gives much information about these tests so that you can intelligently discuss them and their relevance to you with your doctor, your partner, and other family and friends. Many of these tests are fairly routine, like the urine culture to be sure you have no urinary tract infection; others are less commonly done.

Screening Tests

A screening test is a test performed frequently and on people who appear to be well. A good example is the CBC (complete blood count), which helps to identify anemia in pregnancy. The purpose of a screening test is to detect problems early, even before the person is aware of any symptoms, so that these problems can be treated or headed off before they become serious. In the United States, most pregnant women are offered these tests; it is rare for a woman to object to any of these.

A screening test or procedure is not intended to give a diagnosis that is 100 percent accurate every time. Margins of 5 to 10 percent of false positive and false negative results are acceptable statistically in most screening programs. (We'll define false negative and false positive in a moment.) The intent of a *screening* test is simply *to give a fairly high probability that the disease or condition being screened for is or is not there.* On the other hand, a *diagnostic* test is one that tells us definitely whether the suspected disease is present or not. Diagnostic tests are done to find the cause of a particular symptom or to follow up on a positive finding on a screening test. An example of a diagnostic test is an amniocentesis that is done when a screening test has suggested an abnormality in the fetus. (We'll talk about amniocentesis in detail later in this chapter.)

A screening test needs to be both *specific* and *sensitive*. What do we mean by these terms? Being specific means that when the test says that the particular disease or condition isn't present, there is a high probability that it isn't present. Being sensitive means that when the test says that disease *is* present, it is highly probable that the disease or condition is present. However, as we've mentioned, most screening tests are not 100 percent sensitive or specific, and so there will always be some false positive and false negative results with any screening test.

False positive means that the test reads positive—that a particular disease is present—when the person actually does *not* have the disease in question. This is troublesome, because it causes unfounded fear and anxiety, as well as the trauma and cost of further testing; but as long as the percentage of false positives for a test is small, these troublesome consequences are generally considered acceptable. You need to realize before taking any screening test that false positive results can occur.

A *false negative* occurs when the screening test does not pick up the disease but it actually is present. One consequence of false negative test results is that conditions that could be treated go untreated because the test said they weren't there.

So, screening tests are not 100 percent reliable in demonstrating that you have a particular condition. However, in general the screening tests offered to pregnant women have been shown clearly to reduce the incidence and long-term complications of the conditions they have been designed to detect. They can be immensely valuable in protecting and promoting the health of you and your baby.

We say that screening tests are "offered," and it is just that . . . an offer. Women can have good reasons for not taking certain tests. A woman may decline to have an amniocentesis because she knows that she would not choose to abort, even if the baby had Down syndrome or a similar problem. You are under no obligation to accept any of these offered tests. As we've said, some of them do carry risks, and you need to know about the risks in order to make an informed decision. If you don't understand what is going to happen during the test or what it is meant to detect, don't be afraid to ask for more information.

There is often a great deal of societal pressure on women to pursue a "natural" pregnancy and to eschew any medical intervention, including prenatal testing. Nature is an excellent midwife, but she does not always get it right. Until the advent of modern obstetrical techniques, many women and their babies died during pregnancy, in childbirth, or shortly postpartum. These events may be natural, but it is hard to argue that they are better than the alternatives medicine enables. It is natural to walk, but today it is also normal to drive, use trains, and fly in airplanes. Likewise, it is normal, if appropriate in your case, to use whatever technology is needed and available to ensure that you have a healthy baby.

Many of the tests that are offered to women over 35 are no different from the ones offered to younger pregnant women. However, there are some conditions that are more likely to occur in babies of older women, and you need to know something about them.

Down Syndrome

The condition that most increases in frequency among children of women conceiving at older ages is Down syndrome (see Table 2). Hypothetically, if there were a prenatal class for women 41 years old and there were 53 women in the class, one of these women would be likely to have a baby with Down syndrome (and 52 would likely not have an affected baby). The condition causing Down syndrome can and does occur in younger women. The risk in women under 35, however, is lower—around one in 650 (1:650).

Melissa was just 35 when her second son, Hector, was born. She had already had one totally uneventful pregnancy and delivery, and Jorge was 3 years old when Hector was conceived. Since Melissa did not regard herself as an "older" mother she gave no thought to screening for Down syndrome early in her pregnancy. The ultrasound *done at 18 weeks was reported as perfectly normal. At 36 weeks of pregnancy, Melissa went into early labor. The fetal heartbeat slowed alarmingly during labor, and an urgent C-section was performed, with Melissa under general anesthesia. As soon as the doctor saw Hector, he realized that the baby had Down syndrome. When José, Melissa's husband, was introduced to his new son, he was told, "This is your very special son. He is quite healthy, but he will need extra care and attention. We'll talk with you and Melissa more later when she is not so groggy."*

Hector is now 4 years old. Melissa's feelings have evolved over time: "At first I felt shocked that this should have happened. I felt that it was just wrong and unfair. Then, as I held Hector and breastfed him, everything was like it was with Jorge, except that I had to hold him on a pillow to protect the incision on my belly. I won't deny that Hector has made a huge difference in our lives: I didn't go back to work, as I had planned, because Hector needs more of my time and I take him to an early intervention program four days a week to help him develop his potential as fully as possible. He has to see the pediatrician more often than Jorge did, because he needs special checks of his heart, and also he tends to pick up every cough and cold around. But now that I know and love Hector, I am not sure that I would have had a termination in my pregnancy even if I'd known that he was a Down's baby. He is so dear and happy and loving to us all. Certainly having Hector has changed our minds about having more children—we couldn't really cope with any more children now. José has been wonderful, even though this has meant that most of the time he has to work two jobs to support us. His family live near us and they have been very supportive, helping to give us a little time to ourselves and pitching in when it all gets to be too much. I've learned at the early intervention program that having a special needs child often breaks a family up, but we are closer than ever. We are lucky in our support system."

Down syndrome is a genetic disorder. It results when the fertilized egg that develops into a baby contains an extra chromosome (a situation called "trisomy") in its nucleus. In older women, there is an increased chance that two number-21 chromosomes will be

Table 2.   Risk of Down Syndrome with Increasing Age of Mother

Age of Mother at Time of Birth	Risk of Down Syndrome in Baby
35	1/250 or 0.4%
36	1/192 or 0.5%
37	1/149 or 0.7%
38	1/115 or 0.9%
39	1/89 or 1.1%
40	1/69 or 1.4%
41	1/53 or 1.9%
42	1/41 or 2.4%
43	1/31 or 3.2%
44	1/25 or 4.0%
45	1/19 or 5.3%

distributed to the egg, so that when the egg joins with the sperm, the total of number-21 chromosomes is three. This means that all of the cells in the baby's body then contain 47 chromosomes instead of the usual 46. This extra chromosome is responsible for the characteristic clinical features of Down syndrome, which we will describe below. There are a few other, but very rare, chromosomal conditions, also more common in older mothers, and these are detected by the same tests used to detect Down syndrome.

Bernadette was 47 when she began missing her period. She'd spot a little when it was the right time, but there was no real flow. She decided that she was probably going through menopause, and her doctor husband, George, agreed with her. "In fact," he said, "I've noticed that you've been moodier, and menopause could explain that, too." For religious reasons, Bernadette and George have relied on the Billings method of natural family planning, and it had obviously worked well for them, as their youngest child, Tanya, was 12 years old.

Bernadette noticed that she was getting a little rounded belly and joked to her friends about how she was doing all the things the menopause books said: changes in her cycle, emotional swings, and weight gain. "My breasts are sore and I'm awfully tired, too," she observed.

Pregnancy never crossed her mind until the morning that she felt a little bird flutter in her belly—too low to be a skipped heartbeat. Suddenly, her symptoms made sense in a different context, and she phoned her OB/GYN, Dr. McKenna, who had her come in the next day.

An ultrasound, conducted in Dr. McKenna's office, confirmed that Bernadette was 17 weeks pregnant. Because of the much higher risk of Down syndrome in babies born to women in their late forties, Dr. McKenna counseled Bernadette right away about the various tests that were available and suggested that she and George discuss whether they would terminate the pregnancy if there were a strong probability that the baby had Down syndrome.

Bernadette and George's discussion that evening took all of five minutes; a termination of pregnancy would be a great sin in their eyes and there was no negotiating this. Quickly, their discussion turned to a practical matter. How were they going to tell their six children, ranging in age from Tanya at 12 to George Jr., age 24, that their mother was pregnant. Finally, they decided that there was no ideal way to do this; they gathered the family at the customary after-church Sunday brunch and just bluntly announced the forthcoming addition to the family. The reactions varied from Tanya's "Oh, gross!" to George Jr.'s blasé nonchalance, and everything in between.

The remainder of this chapter is about Down syndrome and the prenatal testing for it. We discuss testing for other conditions in Chapter 11.

What Is Down Syndrome?

When an egg and a sperm meet to form the cell that will eventually become a baby, each brings 23 chromosomes from the respective parent, so the baby ends up with 46 chromosomes. In Down syndrome, the baby ends up with 47 chromosomes, because instead of two number-21 chromosomes, there are three (called trisomy 21). Down syndrome is usually easy to recognize in a baby, because it produces characteristic physical features: extra folds of skin (called "epicanthic folds") on the eyes, a short neck, single creases on the sole of the foot and in the palm, short "pinkie" fingers, and thin straight hair. What is less obvious initially is that the baby has a reduced capability for mental and intellectual development and often has heart defects.

The problems that can develop from the diminished mental and intellectual capacity are the principal reasons for offering women early prenatal testing and the possibility of terminating the pregnancy. Most people with Down syndrome will need some type of custodial care for the rest of their lives, be it from parents, other family members, or some other source. This need is a cause of great concern to a mother who will be in her declining years when this child is a young adult. A sensitive and beautifully done French film portrays this problem. George, in *The Eighth Day*, is a young man with Down syndrome whose mother has died and whose sister, with her own husband and young family, is unable to take him in. This film, which will make you laugh and cry in equal measure, tells the story of George's bewilderment at finding himself in a group home and of the tender friendship that develops between him and a stressed and disillusioned insurance executive.

Why Does Down Syndrome Occur?

Trisomy 21 can happen by a random distribution of a third number-21 chromosome in the particular egg from which the baby develops, or by something called translocation, in which one of the two number-21 chromosomes is attached to another chromosome (kind of stuck on it). Translocation can be tested for, and if it is diagnosed, the couple should have genetic counseling to help them know what their particular risk of having a child with Down syndrome would be. Translocations are very rare.

How Do We Screen for Down Syndrome?

What tests are offered to women during their pregnancies in order to detect Down syndrome early enough to have options? The most common screening test offered in the United States at the time of writing is serum screening, a blood test done at 15 to 16 weeks of pregnancy. The duration of the pregnancy is important to the calculations, so if you are not absolutely sure of your dates or don't have very regular cycles, you should have an ultrasound to confirm how many weeks pregnant you are when the blood is taken. Four substances (alpha-fetoprotein, estriol, HCG, and inhibin) are measured in your blood; each of these substances comes from the fetus and/or the placenta. The measurements are then combined with the age you will be when the baby is born, and a computer calculates the statistical risk of your having a baby with Down syndrome, as well as the risk for certain other chromosomal abnormalities. *The test does not definitely answer the question "Does my baby have Down syndrome?"*

May is a 38-year-old woman who has just had her first baby. She elected to have the serum screening test at just over 15 weeks of pregnancy. Her result showed a risk of a Down syndrome baby of 1:737, a much lower risk than her age would imply. May understood that the result was not an absolute guarantee that her baby did not have Down syndrome, but she decided it was sufficiently reassuring for her not to test further by having an amniocentesis. This was a reasonable decision, and May now has a normal and healthy 8 pound daughter.

Heidi is also 38. She underwent serum screening, and her result showed a high risk of a Down's affected child—1:72. Heidi chose to have an amniocentesis and spent sleepless nights until the result came back—showing a baby boy with a normal chromosome count. Heidi finally felt able to announce her pregnancy to family and friends. Heidi's risk assessment—1:72—means that of 72 women with her results it is likely that one will have a baby with Down syndrome and 71 will not. Even though this is not an extremely high risk, it is higher than her age-related risk, which would be 1:115.

Another test, fetal nuchal (neck) translucency (NT) assessment is, as we write, just becoming available in the United States. It has been widely used for some time in the United Kingdom and Australia. What is this test? All developing babies have a layer of fluid on the back of their bodies between the skin and the underlying soft tissue. Because this fluid is translucent, it can be seen and measured on ultrasound imaging. We know that when the thickness of the nuchal translucency is measured between 11 and 14 weeks of pregnancy, an increase in thickness is correlated with a higher risk of Down syndrome, as well as of some rarer chromosomal abnormalities, and with some types of heart problems in the baby.

There are two blood tests that can be done earlier, in the first trimester. These are beta-HCG (human chorionic gonadotropin) and PAPP-A (pregnancy-associated plasma protein A). While these blood tests are not sufficiently predictive on their own, their results can be combined with that of the fetal nuchal translucency and with the mother's age to calculate the woman's risk of having a baby with Down syndrome, as the more-established serum screening does. By this testing method, a low risk is more than one in three hundred, a high risk, less than one in three hundred. The blood tests are usually done at around 10 weeks followed by the NT measurement at 12 weeks. Because this combination of blood tests and NT assessment is done before 12 or 13 weeks of pregnancy, women with high-risk results can decide whether or not to have diagnostic testing (described in the next section) at 13 weeks.

There are two important things to understand about nuchal translucency/blood testing done at 10 to 12 weeks of pregnancy:

- A normal or low-risk result does not guarantee that the baby will be normal, but it does suggest that Down syndrome or a heart problem are unlikely.
- An abnormal or high-risk result does not mean that the baby is abnormal, but it does suggest that further investigations be done if the parents want to have a definite answer in order to be able to consider abortion or make arrangements to care for a child with special needs.

Within the high-risk group, more than half of the women deliver babies that are perfectly normal, as is the case for women with high-risk results on the 15–16 week serum screening.

It has been estimated that the NT ultrasound alone will identify 80 percent of those babies with abnormalities who are tested and that the blood tests will add a further 10 percent of identifications, but there will be false positives as well.

Your fetal nuchal translucency ultrasound should be done by a well-trained sonographer—a technician who has received specialized training and certification in ultrasound techniques—or a radiologist or fetal medicine specialist who has this training and accreditation. You should feel free to ask your doctor or the local medical society if the technicians where you will be tested meet these criteria.

Ideally, ultrasound and serum screening are done in conjunction with counseling about the different screening options and about the limitations of the various tests and how these factors apply to you personally. The results of the ultrasound will be relayed to your referring doctor, who will discuss them with you.

Because most children are born to women under age 35, the vast majority of children with Down syndrome are born to women younger than 35. The screening tests can be done on any pregnant woman, regardless of age, and it is anticipated that, over the next few years, offering them to all pregnant women will become routine practice.

As mentioned, it is vitally important that your length of gestation be known when ordering any of these tests. If you are unsure of the date of your last period, if you have irregular cycles, or if you have gotten pregnant while using some form of hormonal birth control, you should have a "dating" ultrasound soon after your positive pregnancy test. This is a very accurate way to determine how far along you are (and whether there might be more than one baby). The beating heart can also tell us that the fetus is living, or "viable." At this early stage, not much other information can be learned.

DIAGNOSTIC TESTS

Diagnostic tests may be offered to any woman who has had a "high risk" result on the screening tests we've just described. A woman may opt to have a diagnostic test without previous screens. She may make this decision because she is over 35, has had a previously affected pregnancy, or has had a family member with Down syndrome or one of the rarer chromosomal abnormalities. Both of the diagnostic tests currently available are invasive in that they involve taking some of the baby's cells from the mother's body. Doing this obviously involves some risks for both the mother and the baby.

CVS

Chorionic villous sampling (CVS) is done at about 12 weeks of pregnancy and involves passing a needle up through the cervical canal into the developing placenta to take a small sample of the tissue. The passage of the needle is guided by ultrasound to make sure that a good sample is obtained and to keep the needle away from the developing baby. Some testing centers do the procedure through the abdominal wall, again guided by ultrasound. Usually, the mother is given some light sedation or an analgesic (pain killer). There is a small risk that miscarriage will result from CVS—from as low as 0.5 percent to as high as 3 percent, depending on who is doing the test, and where—but the test has the advantage of giving a quick answer: the fetal cells are examined and the chromosomal makeup determined within 48 to 72 hours.

The biggest practical advantage of CVS is that if abnormalities are detected and the parents decide to abort, a termination at this stage is a much simpler and less traumatic event for the woman than later in the pregnancy. Disadvantages include that occasionally not enough cells are obtained by the procedure to give an accurate result, and occasionally a condition called mosaicism is present, in which there is a chromosomal difference between the cells in the placental tissue and the cells of the developing baby to whom that placenta is attached, and the correct chromosomal result is not obtained. Overall, however, CVS is more than 99 percent accurate.

After a CVS there may be a small amount of vaginal bleeding or discharge. Anything more than a very little bit should be reported to your doctor.

Amniocentesis

Amniocentesis is usually done later in the pregnancy—between 15 and 18 weeks of gestation. It can detect the presence of many kinds of genetic disorders. It can also identify the sex of the fetus.

Ana, *to whom you were introduced earlier, is typical of many older women in her feelings and decisions about prenatal testing for Down syndrome. She had serum testing done when she was close to 16 weeks, because she wanted to be reassured by good results, which she got. But, because the blood tests did not give her a definite diagnostic result, she also opted for an amniocentesis. She chose it over CVS because the risk of miscarriage from the procedure is lower. Fortunately, Ana's results showed a normal chromosome count in her baby—and she decided against learning the baby's sex from the amniocentesis.*

On the day of the test, Ana took Kenyon along to hold her hand, and she was very glad he was there. She'd already read (about fifteen times) the information she'd been given about what would happen. When she performed the amniocentesis, Dr. Ramsay first put some local anesthetic into the skin of Ana's belly to make the procedure more comfortable. Ana was aware of pressure but no real pain. Using ultrasound to guide her, Dr. Ramsay passed a long needle through Ana's abdominal wall into one of the pools of amniotic fluid that surrounds and protects the baby. Ultrasound guidance allowed Dr. Ramsay to avoid the baby and the placenta—she could literally see where she was placing the needle. About 20 ml of fluid (about 4 teaspoonfuls) were drawn off and sent to the lab for testing.

In most cases, the fluid contains enough cells shed by the baby for a culture to grow from the cells; the culture is then examined for a chromosome count. This process takes about two to three weeks. A new technique, fluorescent in-situ hybridization (FISH), is quicker, having a turnaround time of 24 hours. In this technique, fluorescent-labeled DNA probes are used to "attach" to specific chromosomal areas, enabling quicker identification. FISH is fairly accurate in identifying trisomy 21 (Down syndrome), but the standard methods of typing are still the gold standard.

Often if a woman is relaxed about the procedure no anesthetic is needed, but you should have a choice in this matter. After the procedure, it is generally recommended that you take it easy for a few hours, so plan the rest of your day accordingly. The puncture mark on your abdomen is simply covered with an ordinary adhesive bandage. If you have any bleeding or leaking of clear fluid from your vagina after the test, you should report it at once to your doctor.

Sometimes amniocentesis shows a chromosomal abnormality other than Down syndrome. It may be another kind of trisomy, for example trisomy 13 or 18, both of which combine distinctive physical characteristics with intellectual disability, just as trisomy 21 does. In these disorders, the same kinds of factors will affect your decision to terminate the pregnancy or not and what kind of life you and the child might have. Some people born with chromosomal abnormalities can lead ordinary lives and have normal intellectual capacity, although some will require medication and treatment in childhood. This group includes abnormalities of the sex chromosomes, the X and Y chromosomes. The most common of these conditions is Turner's syndrome, in which one X chromosome is absent. All of these children are girls. To accomplish normal growth and development they require hormone treatment. They may also have heart problems that will require surgery, but they are intellectually normal. Should your amniocentesis result in a diagnosis of one of these conditions, just as with Down syndrome you will need to discuss your situation fully with your doctors. There are also support groups to provide advice and help, some of which are listed in the Resources section at the back of this book.

Responding to Test Results

If your test results indicate that you have a fetus with Down syndrome or some other identifiable abnormality and you come to the decision to terminate the pregnancy, you should know how that would be accomplished—and you should know this before deciding whether or not to have the tests. The procedures for terminating a pregnancy are described in Chapter 13.

Facing the birth of a child with Down syndrome is an enormous challenge. In deciding what to do, you should seek whatever assistance and support you need. You are entitled to sympathetic, nonjudgmental, and accurate advice from your health care providers. Here are three rather different stories of people confronted with this situation.

Joan was 41 when she unexpectedly became pregnant in the course of a fairly casual relationship. Joan is divorced and had never been pregnant—and she felt quite guarded about the possibility of continuing the pregnancy. Joan is a math graduate and works in an engineering firm; she could see that the risks of having a baby with genetic abnormalities were statistically greater than the risks of miscarriage from CVS, and she chose to have the testing done. She decided she would not allow herself to look at the ultrasound images of her baby during either her early ultrasound or the CVS. When her report showed Down syndrome, Joan opted at once for an abortion under a general anesthetic. But she was surprised at how much sadness she felt afterwards. She was glad to have the help from the clinic's counselor, and she visited the counselor several times. Joan has many friends, but she had not wanted to confide this particular difficulty to any of them.

Sarita and Bill have been married for 17 years and have five healthy sons, ranging in age from 16 down to 6. They are a very religious family and live their beliefs in their everyday life; one of those beliefs is that any artificial contraception is wrong. They had used natural family planning successfully for many years, but when Sarita was 41, she unexpectedly conceived. She and Bill declined any of the prenatal tests that screen for Down syndrome because termination was simply not an option for them. At 18 weeks, Sarita did have an ultrasound that showed some features in the baby's neck and fingers that suggested Down syndrome. It also suggested an abnormality in the baby's heart. After careful discussion with the doctors and a counselor, and hours of prayer with their priest, Sarita and Bill decided to do nothing more and let nature take its course. At 35 weeks, Sarita went into labor and soon gave birth to a daughter, who was baptized immediately and named Aniella. Aniella did have Down syndrome; she also had a severe heart condition. When she was just a few hours old, she died peacefully in her mother's arms, with her daddy and her big brothers standing close by. At least they each had had a chance to see and hold her. Sarita still grieves for her daughter but does not regret the choices that she and her family made. "We lost her, but at least we knew her first, however briefly."

Alison *conceived for the first time at age 39. She was successful in her career and had set a five-year plan with her partner, Len. This plan involved pregnancy at about age 39 with the resultant birth of a single — preferably female — child. Alison felt sure that the baby would be perfect because she was herself in such good health and because she had so quickly and easily conceived.*

Alison knew she wanted to have an amniocentesis at 16 weeks, and since she had already planned for this test, she decided against the earlier screening tests for Down syndrome. She never even dreamed that the amniocentesis results might be positive — the chances were so much against it, 90 to one. She was devastated when her doctor called her in about two weeks later to tell her that she was carrying a baby with Down syndrome. She was angry and told him that there had to be an error.

Alison and Len struggled with what to do, but after a couple of days agreed that they were in no position to take care of a special needs child. Len was terrified about what would become of her or him as they, the parents, aged and could no longer adequately provide daily care. They concurred that Alison should have a termination.

It is very difficult for any of us to envisage ourselves in predicaments such as we've outlined. And indeed, despite the higher incidence of chromosomal abnormalities in older women, the statistics are still in your favor. Most women over 35 who conceive, indeed most women over 45 who conceive, do *not* have a baby with Down syndrome. At 35 the risk is 1:250, meaning 249 chances out of 250 that the baby will not be affected; at 45, 1 in 19 is affected, and 18 are unaffected.

If you should face this difficult situation, you deserve sympathetic and professional care from all your health care providers, and you deserve adequate pain management if you elect termination. If you are not comfortable with the care or treatment you are getting, you may want to change health care providers. As you can imagine, a late termination is even more emotionally devastating and physically traumatic to a woman than an earlier termination. It is extremely important that you and your partner have plenty of information and set aside enough time to make your decision if you are faced with this situation. You may want to do the same even as you contemplate getting pregnant.

Chapter 11

——— ∿ ———

Prenatal Tests

Prenatal tests are done during the pregnancy to assess the health of the mother and the developing fetus. If any abnormality is detected, early knowledge of it gives time to consider options and correct the problem if possible. Which tests are offered varies a little from one region to another, but certain blood and urine tests are common everywhere.

A summary descriptive list of the tests discussed here and others, along with a chronological list showing at what point in a pregnancy they are performed, can be found in Appendix H of this book.

ULTRASOUND

Ultrasonography is a painless, nonintrusive way to see into the human body. Very high frequency sound waves are used to create images. Ultrasonograms are now routinely offered in most medical centers. The person performing the scan should be accredited and experienced. During pregnancy, the test is generally done at some point between 18 and 20 weeks. Often the ultrasonogram can be turned into a video (you may need to bring your own tape), but nearly always you will be given some still pictures to take home with you.

For most women this is an exciting and interesting experience that they wish to share with their partners. The main point of the test, however, is to examine the fetus to check that certain organs and systems appear normal. Are the baby's head, brain, face, heart, lungs, stomach, kidneys, bladder, and limbs developing as expected? Is further testing indicated? It is usually possible to tell what sex the baby is, but you should be asked in advance whether or not you want to learn this information before the birth. Speak up if you want to wait.

Clearly, if you are to have a week 18 scan, you need to know when you will be at week 18. Scans done too early will not be able to see enough detail to be useful, and if a scan is done too late and a major abnormality is identified, there will be fewer options for dealing with the situation. It is wise to have your dates checked with an earlier, "dating" ultrasound scan, which will also tell you whether or not you are carrying twins and will identify the location of the placenta.

After the ultrasound done at 18 to 20 weeks, a small number of parents will receive the unwelcome news that their baby has an abnormality. In the previous chapter we told you about Sarita, whose ultrasound indicated the presence of Down syndrome with a heart abnormality. She and her husband decided to continue with her pregnancy.

Mara is a woman of 36 who had a routine ultrasound scan at 19 weeks in her first pregnancy. A severe fetal heart abnormality was discovered. After much discussion with several doctors, who confirmed that no surgery would be able to correct the defect after the child was born, Mara decided on termination of the pregnancy. Currently she is pregnant again, and this time the ultrasound does not show any problems. However, a normal-looking scan does not guarantee a perfect baby; ultrasound technicians can only report on what they see on their screens.

The week 18 ultrasound can also pick up on problems that are totally compatible with normal living but for which the baby will require some treatment, possibly surgery at or soon after birth.

Claudia and David's son Josh was diagnosed with a cleft lip and palate on Claudia's week 18 scan. Well before Josh arrived, the couple read up on the condition, met and talked to the pediatric surgeon who subsequently cared for Josh, and learned how to feed him expressed breast milk in the weeks before his first surgery because he would not be able to nurse.

When an ultrasound reveals a condition that can be treated at birth, alterations in plans for the birth may be suggested, so that the birth can take place close to a center where specialized pediatric surgery is available.

Blood Tests

Blood tests done during pregnancy usually include the complete blood count (CBC), blood glucose, blood type, tests for Rh factor and other antibodies that may be present in the blood, rubella immunity status, hepatitis B and C immunity status, and RPR test for syphilis. HIV testing is encouraged, but it is not routinely done.

Complete Blood Count

CBC is done particularly to be sure that a woman is not anemic. Anemia, especially iron-deficiency anemia, is a relatively common problem in women even when not pregnant. If anemia is diagnosed during pregnancy, correcting the condition as early as possible is important. The red blood cells contain hemoglobin, the substance by which oxygen is transported in the blood and delivered to the developing baby as well as to the mother's vital organs. If you don't have enough hemoglobin, you are anemic. In pregnancy there is an increase in the number of red blood cells, but there is an even greater increase in the plasma (the milky fluid in which the red and white cells float), so the proportion of hemoglobin in the blood becomes diluted. This means that pregnant women normally have lower hemoglobin levels than nonpregnant women. During the first two trimesters (up to about 28 weeks), a woman is considered to be anemic if her hemoglobin falls below 11 grams per deciliter (g/dL); and in the last three months, she is anemic if it falls below 10.5. When these levels fall, we recommend treatment with iron supplements in addition to the supplement the mother is already getting in the prenatal vitamins she should be taking. Sometimes anemia due to folic acid deficiency or vitamin B_{12} deficiency may be indicated by the blood smear.

Blood Group

Testing for blood group is done primarily in case you should need a blood transfusion around the time of birth. Although few women need a transfusion during delivery, it is something your doctors should be prepared for. Occasionally a woman has some unusual antibodies in her blood, and these are screened for so that compatible blood will be available should she need it.

Rh Factor

Rh or Rhesus factor is important. Being Rhesus positive (Rh+) simply means that you have a protein called the Rhesus factor attached to your red blood cells. A person who does not have Rhesus factor is said to be Rh negative. All blood transfusion services in the United States now make sure that Rh-negative people do not receive Rh-positive blood, but a woman can become pregnant with a baby who is Rh positive. This can happen if the baby's father is Rh positive, and since 85 percent of white Americans, 95 percent of African Americans, and 99 percent of Asian Americans are Rh positive, this is quite likely.

If during the pregnancy or labor some of the baby's red blood cells enter the mother's bloodstream, the mother's body may start making antibodies to Rhesus-positive red blood cells. In a later pregnancy, again with a Rhesus-positive baby, these antibodies may cross the placenta and destroy the baby's red blood cells, causing the baby to become increasingly anemic and possibly die. In other words, the first pregnancy can act to sensitize the mother so that later pregnancies are put at risk.

Until a few decades ago, Rh-negative women often lost babies because of this incompatibility. Today this rarely happens, because we screen mothers ahead of time and treat those at risk with small doses of antibody before their own systems begin to manufacture permanent antibodies to the Rh-positive red cells. This treatment has revolutionized the care of Rh disease in newborns, which until the 1970s was a major cause of death in babies. Now the antibody, known commercially as Rhogam, is given to Rhesus-negative women after they give birth to Rh-positive babies, during pregnancy if there is any bleeding or any procedure that may cause a transfer of red blood cells from the baby to the mother, and preventatively at weeks 28 and 34 of pregnancy.

There are some other much less common antibodies that can affect a baby in the same way as Rh antibodies, and these are routinely screened for, too.

German Measles

"Rubella antibody titers" measure the levels of antibodies against German measles (rubella). Having rubella in the first weeks of pregnancy can cause severe birth defects in the baby, including hearing and vision defects and heart problems. The advent of a vaccine against rubella has made these tragedies virtually unheard of today. This vaccine is usually given in childhood. Once in a while, a woman will have inadequate rubella immunity. If she is already pregnant, she will have to protect herself against exposure during pregnancy and then be immunized after the baby is born.

Hepatitis B

Hepatitis B is a very serious, very infectious blood-borne disease. All parents of newborn infants are now advised to have the child vaccinated against it, and we are hopeful that this policy of universal immunization will eradicate the illness. We screen pregnant women to identify those who are immune to hepatitis B, either because they have been vaccinated or because they have experienced a mild case of the infection and developed their own antibodies, and those who contracted the infection earlier in their lives and are still infectious because it has not completely cleared their bodies. The babies born to women still harboring the disease are at greater risk of contracting hepatitis B in the few months after birth, so they are given globulin, which protects them against such infection, and are vaccinated.

Hepatitis C

Although hepatitis C is most common in drug users and sex workers, good public health policy dictates that we screen all pregnant women, and many hospitals and clinics do. Ask what the practice is at your hospital or clinic. Because hepatitis C can be transmitted to the baby without the mother even realizing she is infected, women need to know as soon as possible if the infection is present, so that they can get counseling and treatment.

Syphilis

The RPR (rapid plasmin regain) test and similar tests screen for syphilis. They are done routinely because the effects of this sexually transmitted disease, which can be contracted by the baby in the womb, are devastating. Treatment with antibiotics is effective, but the bacterium needs to be identified in the mother before treatment is given. Laboratories automatically confirm positive results with more specific diagnostic tests, to be sure.

Diabetes

Blood glucose screening is done early in pregnancy by many hospitals and clinics because gestational diabetes (diabetes first occurring during pregnancy) is becoming more common. The sooner the mother is treated, using diet and/or insulin, the better for the baby. This test and the reasons for it are explained in detail in Chapter 7.

HIV/AIDS

Screening pregnant women for HIV (human immunodeficiency virus) has caused much controversy. The current public policy in most regions of the United States is to encourage voluntary screening for HIV but not to require it; check with your doctor about the practices in your particular community and state. From the baby's point of view, it is important to diagnose maternal HIV infection before delivery, because we now have drugs that will prevent transmission of the virus to the baby. It has also been shown to be safer to deliver the baby by Cesarean section, to further decrease the risk of transmission to the baby.

URINALYSIS

Urine is examined for protein (to check for kidney disease), glucose (looking for diabetes), and blood; a culture is grown from the specimen, by adding it to a special growth medium, to see whether bacteria grow. Any urinary tract infection needs to be detected early, even if it isn't causing symptoms, because a mild infection can become more severe later in pregnancy and can cause kidney damage and increase the risk of premature labor.

A midstream specimen of urine is routinely examined at the first prenatal visit. A midstream specimen is obtained by first passing some urine into the toilet bowl, then catching some in the jar provided to you. Given the size of the jar, this can be a difficult anatomical exercise (we speak from experience). There is a reason for doing the procedure this way. The first urine that is passed may be contaminated with bacteria and skin cells from the skin at the opening of the urethra (the passage from the bladder to the outside), but the midstream specimen more accurately shows whether any infection is present internally. (You may also be provided with an antiseptic wipe to cleanse the vulva before producing the urine specimen.)

TUBERCULOSIS SKIN TEST

In areas of relatively high tuberculosis risk, a PPD (purified protein derivative) skin test is used to screen expectant mothers for TB. This test is not universally applied in pregnancy but should be done on women in certain populations or geographic regions at greater risk—for example, women living on American Indian reservations, inner city residents, and those who are occupationally exposed to patients with TB.

Your doctor should discuss the results of your prenatal testing with you at your next visit, and any abnormalities should be dealt with as soon as possible.

Chapter 12

————— ❧ —————

Miscarriage

Between 15 and 20 percent of all pregnancies end in miscarriage (sometimes called spontaneous abortion). This means that 1 woman in 5 to 6 will have a single miscarriage; 1 in 30 of those who have a first miscarriage will miscarry the next pregnancy as well. A woman who has a third miscarriage in a row is said to have "recurrent miscarriage" or "recurrent pregnancy loss." In a younger woman, some investigations into the cause of this situation are usually done after the third miscarriage; in an older woman, testing may be appropriate after the second.

The main reason for miscarriage is that the embryo is abnormal in some way; often the problem is chromosomal. Miscarriage is "nature's way" of keeping such embryos from developing further. Recurrent miscarriage in a woman is not necessarily caused by a particular abnormality or the same abnormality each time, so testing the fetus is rarely helpful in determining the cause or preventing recurrences.

Miscarriage generally occurs between 6 and 12 weeks of pregnancy. It usually starts with some vaginal bleeding, with or without pain. The pain that follows often feels like menstrual cramps; the uterus is contracting to expel the pregnancy. If you feel such cramping, miscarriage is likely. Bleeding without pain may settle down and be followed by a normal pregnancy.

Miscarriage can also occur later in pregnancy (up to 24 weeks, the time at which a baby may be capable of surviving in the world). Like earlier miscarriage, it may commence with bleeding followed by pains that lead to the expulsion of the fetus. Sometimes later miscarriage occurs because the placenta has become detached from the wall of the uterus, sometimes because the mother has an infection either in the uterus or somewhere else in the body, and some-times it happens for no obvious reason.

In some cases, late miscarriage may be related to previous ab-dominal operations, such as cone biopsy for cervical precancer (see Chapter 8) or other surgeries that have caused the cervix to be "incompetent" at holding the pregnancy in place. Late miscar-riage of this type often starts with painless leakage of amniotic fluid vaginally, followed by some contractions, leading to expulsion of the fetus. There may not be much bleeding or pain. Hoping to prevent late miscarriage in a woman known to have cervical incompetence, some doctors place a stitch around the cervix to hold the pregnancy in place, but there is debate as to how effective this intervention is.

If you have any vaginal bleeding during the early weeks of preg-nancy, visit your doctor. You may be examined vaginally, to see if your cervix has started to open, a sign that the pregnancy is not continuing and that miscarriage is inevitable. You may also have an ultrasound, which will either show that pregnancy is continu-ing and the fetus is alive (the fetal heart is seen to be beating) or confirm that miscarriage is occurring.

If the bleeding is heavy, a D&C (dilation and curettage) will usually be performed, under anesthesia or sedation, removing pla-cental and fetal tissue. This stops the bleeding. The uterus begins to shrink, and over about four weeks it returns to its normal size and shape. After four to six weeks periods return. Sometimes a drug to stop bleeding (ergonovine) is also given.

In the majority of miscarriages, bleeding is slight. The pregnan-cy is gradually passed vaginally, and over about a week's time the bleeding stops. Many women are happy not to have had surgical intervention. Infection is a potential problem; if your temperature goes up you will need antibiotics, and a D&C may be necessary to remove remaining tissue from the pregnancy that has become infected.

Occasionally when bleeding occurs very early in pregnancy and an ultrasound is done to find out why, the test fails to detect a fetal heartbeat simply because the pregnancy is too early. In this case it is usual to wait up to a week and repeat the ultrasound, unless bleeding becomes heavier and it is clear that miscarriage is going to occur. To repeat, some slight bleeding in very early pregnancy is not necessarily an indication that the pregnancy won't continue normally.

Miscarriage is an event that causes a great deal of sorrow to women, and a woman who has a miscarriage will need good support. Grief over a miscarriage in early pregnancy, even an unplanned pregnancy, can be particularly hard to bear, because few people will be aware that you were pregnant. Since you would have to reveal the pregnancy and miscarriage both, you may not wish to tell anyone beyond your partner and immediate family or friends. The grief is especially acute when a long-desired pregnancy had finally been achieved, as is not infrequently the case for older women. The feeling of loss can be accompanied by a sense of failure, even though miscarriage is not anyone's fault. Work or normal exercise or having sex does not cause miscarriage. Doing those things, even after an episode of vaginal bleeding (a "threatened" miscarriage), is perfectly all right. Definitely recommended in a continuing pregnancy or in a pregnancy after previous miscarriage is supplemental folic acid, which we mention elsewhere.

INVESTIGATION OF RECURRENT MISCARRIAGE

Whether to do investigative tests and how much to search for the cause of recurrent miscarriage is up to you and your doctor. Causes that may be tested for include:

- Chromosomal abnormalities in one of the parents
- Thyroid disease
- Syphilis (an uncommon cause)
- Autoimmune conditions, such as lupus
- Raised levels of certain antibodies, in particular what are called anticardiolipin antibodies
- Abnormalities of the shape of the uterus
- Infections of the cervix and vagina

The mother or the father may have a chromosomal defect that is not evident but can be passed to the developing baby (such as the translocation discussed in Chapter 10). Women who have had a threatened or definite miscarriage routinely have their blood tested to determine the blood group, and receive Rhogam if they are Rh negative. An ultrasound scan or examination with a hysteroscope will reveal abnormalities in the shape of the uterus. Among infections that might be found, a common one caused by *Gardnerella* bacteria is suspected of causing recurrent miscarriage. The connection has not been proven, but it is reasonable to treat bacterial vaginosis with antibiotics if it is present.

How Soon after a Miscarriage to Become Pregnant Again?

If you have had a D&C, you may want to get back to feeling more normal before you try again to conceive. Most women wait one or two cycles at least before trying again, but there is no overwhelming medical reason not to start right away if you wish.

If you conceive again immediately after a miscarriage, without having a period, ultrasound can be used to date the beginning of the pregnancy. The ultrasound will also give good evidence as to whether the new pregnancy is continuing safely.

Chapter 13

―――― ❦ ――――

Termination of Pregnancy

We would be sugarcoating the facts and failing to provide all the information that a woman may need if we pretended that all pregnancies in women over age 35 are planned and wanted. Most are, and most women who do *not* want to be pregnant take appropriate precautions to prevent pregnancy. But, even sterilization and the best contraceptive measures sometimes fail. Also, as we discuss at some length in Chapter 10, early screening for abnormalities in the fetus may reveal serious problems, in the face of which termination is an option. Occasionally an older woman who had simply not realized she was pregnant until well into the pregnancy will find herself having to contemplate a late abortion.

Many women who find themselves unexpectedly pregnant are initially shaken by the situation but then decide that they can, after all, look forward to and welcome the new arrival. However, not all can do this, and their choices need to be honored, too. Geraldine comes to mind.

Geraldine is in her early forties and has a very comfortable life. She runs her own business, travels widely, and has an active social life, with friends of both sexes. For a long time, she has known that she does not want to marry or have children. She is sexually active but is careful to practice contraception.

A couple of years ago, Geraldine missed a menstrual period. At first, she thought maybe it was the onset of an early menopause, but then she began vomiting after breakfast. A home pregnancy test confirmed her suspicions. For about six hours she entertained the notion of motherhood, but then she had to admit to herself that she could not do it. Geraldine went to a private clinic and had a termination of the pregnancy. Surprised when she afterward grieved for the loss, she arranged to go in for a sterilization the following month. She did not want to go through that experience again. Although she still harbors some regrets, she knows that she made the right choice for her.

Other abortions are in response to test results indicating severe abnormalities in the fetus.

Alison and Len, whose story is introduced in Chapter 10, conceived a very planned and wanted child when Alison was 39. Amniocentesis at 16 weeks confirmed that the fetus had Down syndrome. Having decided that they could not provide a lifetime of care for a person with special needs, they reluctantly elected to terminate the pregnancy. Several hours of vaginal suppositories ensued, followed by a "mini-labor" and the expulsion of a female fetus with Down syndrome. The doctor and nursing staff were very kind, and Alison had adequate physical pain relief during her procedure.

Their families went out of their way to be supportive, but both Alison and Len felt guilty and depressed for months afterward and were afraid to try for another pregnancy. Finally, on a trip away, to try to help deal with their grief, they conceived again—unintentionally. Fortunately, CVS testing at 12 weeks revealed this to be a normal pregnancy, and their healthy son, Damon, was born six months later. Only then did Alison and Len really feel they were beginning to heal.

SURGICAL ABORTION

Termination of a pregnancy after 9 weeks but before 14 weeks can be done by suction curettage (a D&C, dilation and curettage). The cervix is dilated under either local or general anesthesia, and a suction device is passed through the opened cervix. This device removes the fetal and placental tissue. Sometimes dilation of the cervix is assisted by taking oral medication before the procedure or by inserting into the canal of the cervix suppositories that swell and assist in its opening.

This procedure is usually done in an outpatient surgery clinic and is completed in about 20 minutes. You are able to go home soon afterwards. Bleeding and discharge following the procedure can last up to about three weeks. To have a termination safely performed by this technique, you must be not more than 14 weeks advanced in your pregnancy.

MEDICAL ABORTION

As the name implies, "medical" abortions are brought about by taking medications that end the pregnancy. These procedures simulate natural miscarriage. They are used very early in pregnancy—before 9 weeks—for reasons of privacy and because they have few side effects at that stage. Medical abortion is also preferred after 14 weeks, as the uterus grows larger and there would be a greater risk of bleeding, infection, and damage to other organs in a surgical abortion.

In a medical termination, drugs are given to stimulate the uterus to contract. These medications are administered by pill, injection, vaginal gels, or pessaries (vaginal suppositories), depending on the drug. The length of time it takes the drugs to work and the duration of the resultant labor and expulsion process vary but tend to be a matter of hours. The fetus and the placenta are expelled through the vagina. The placenta may need to be removed under anesthesia because it has not separated and delivered with the fetus.

Two of the medications used are mifepristone and methotrexate. Mifepristone, or RU-486, has been called the abortion pill. It was first licensed in France in 1988 and was approved for use in the United States in September 2000. It acts by blocking the hormone progesterone, which is necessary to sustain pregnancy. Ninety-five percent of women who take mifepristone will abort within one week, usually within hours. Methotrexate is better known for its use in treating cancer and autoimmune diseases, but it is also known to stop the implantation of the fetus. It is usually given by injection, although it may be given orally. It is not as effective or efficient as mifepristone.

A few days after taking either mifepristone or methotrexate, a woman may be given a second drug, misoprostol, which causes the uterus to contract and empty. The woman will usually experience cramping and bleeding that may be heavier than her normal period.

Sometimes, a combination of methods—gradual opening of the cervix using drugs and then dilation and curettage of the uterus—is used in termination of a later pregnancy. Occasionally, a technique called hysterotomy is used for termination of a later pregnancy. A hysterotomy, done under anesthetic, is very similar to a Cesarean section. It may be used if a woman has had previous surgeries on her uterus, such as previous C-sections or surgery for fibroids, putting it at greater risk of rupture if contractions are artificially stimulated.

Terminations after 14 weeks are done in the United States and other countries, but the laws controlling and limiting the procedure vary from place to place.

AFTER THE PROCEDURE

Earlier termination does not produce a baby that is recognizable as such, but later termination does. It is your right to see and hold your baby, take photos, and have a funeral or other ceremony. It is equally your right to do none of these things. These difficult situations trigger deep grief and often feelings of blame directed at yourself or your partner—even though nobody is "to blame." It is natural to grieve and you need to be lovingly supported during this time. You may need the help of a trained counselor. Make use of all the resources available to you.

Termination of a pregnancy, especially in the later weeks, is an emotionally distressing and physiologically stressful experience for a woman. The circumstances that lead her to end her pregnancy can in themselves be disturbing. Her decision should be respected, and she should be given all the support she needs as she goes through this ordeal. The National Abortion Federation provides support and information for women faced with this difficult choice, at their hotline, 1-800-772-9100, and on their Web site, www.pro-choice.org.

Chapter 14

——— ❧ ———

Lifestyle during Pregnancy

HEALTH AND DIET

These days, pregnant women can continue their lives much as before pregnancy, but extra attention does need to be given to optimizing your health during this important time. You are probably sick of hearing that you are eating for two, but it is true. As a rule of thumb, if enough nutrients are not supplied for both you and the baby, the baby will get the best ones. This is why the old adage "a tooth for every baby," referring to the leaching of calcium from the mother's body, was true, and still is true in impoverished societies. Today, most women in developed countries can avoid the toll pregnancy can take on a mother's body by getting good nutrition. This is not the time for fad diets or attempts at weight loss. A good balanced diet is the key, and it is possible for vegetarians as well as nonvegetarians. If you are following a specific diet plan, whether it be for health problems or philosophical reasons, ask a dietitian how to fit all the nutritional elements you are going to need into your own specific dietary limitations.

In your balanced diet, include high-quality carbohydrates, such as fruits, vegetables, and whole grains. If you have gluten sensitivity, you can still eat rice, and brown rice is a good source of fiber and B vitamins, as well as carbohydrate calories. Include protein in your diet; if you are vegetarian, you can use beans, nuts, and seeds, as well as dairy products and eggs if you are not vegan. It is not a bad idea for vegetarians to have your doctor check your B_{12} levels, so that you can supplement with this vitamin if necessary.

Try to avoid eating a lot of processed foods, including white breads, cereals, crackers, and snack foods. Instead, satisfy your hunger with fruits, vegetables, and protein as much as possible. Be sure to include some oils in your diet; good ones are olive, canola, flax seed, and walnut. These are sources of good fatty acids that both you and your baby need.

A common question asked by pregnant women is "How much weight should I gain?" We know what weight gain is optimal for women, based on their body mass index prior to becoming pregnant. See Appendix C to easily determine your body mass index (BMI). The Institute of Medicine makes the following recommendations:

Underweight women (BMI less than 19.8) should gain 28 to 40 lb.
Average-weight women (BMI 19.8 to 26) should gain 25 to 35 lb.
Overweight women (BMI greater than 26) should gain 15 to 25 lb.

These ranges of weight gain have been associated with optimal newborn weights.

There are a few foods and supplements about which you need to be cautious. Unless your doctor specifically recommends other vitamins, stick to a prenatal multivitamin, and calcium and iron if prescribed, while you are pregnant. Certain other supplements may be problematic, notably vitamin A, iodine, and vitamin C in large amounts. Your diet and prenatal multivitamin contain all you will need of these nutrients while you are pregnant.

Fish, while it is a wonderful source of protein and good fatty acids, should be eaten judiciously in pregnancy because many fish are polluted with mercury and other environmental toxins. While pregnant or breastfeeding, enjoy cod, pollock, and haddock often, and eat salmon, flounder, and sole no more than once weekly. Avoid tuna, bluefish, catfish, striped bass, shark, and swordfish, however, because they are too likely to contain high levels of contaminants. Also avoid the sushi bar while you are pregnant: raw fish may be contaminated with bacteria. Freshwater fish can be a problem; in many areas their levels of contaminants are too high for you to safely eat them. Since this situation varies by locale, check with your state department of health or the dietitian at the local hospital.

Caffeine is definitely best taken in smaller amounts during pregnancy, no more each day than the equivalent of one and a half cups of brewed coffee. Consuming more than 500 milligrams of caffeine per day has been linked to miscarriage, and drinking more than four cups of brewed caffeinated coffee a day may increase the risk of stillbirth. Conveniently, many women find that an aversion to coffee and/or tea comes along with the first signs of pregnancy. See Appendix D for a listing of the caffeine content of various beverages and types of chocolate. Be aware that some over-the-counter medications contain caffeine. If you are not already a conscientious label reader, become one.

Just in case you didn't know—any form of alcoholic beverage is out. In the first trimester, alcohol can damage the developing fetus. Later in your pregnancy, you might allow a single toast for your wedding anniversary or birthday, but don't extend this to the birthdays and celebrations of all your friends! As with coffee and tea, a lot of women find that they develop an aversion to alcohol during pregnancy.

Smoking is a bad thing to do during pregnancy. It can retard the growth of your baby in your womb. "Small-for-date" babies have a multitude of problems after birth and in later life, and knowing that smoking can cause low birth weight should give you the necessary will power to quit if you have this habit.

Heightened sexual receptivity may accompany the hormones of pregnancy, especially during the middle months of pregnancy; this is a delight to many and a compensation for the nausea, tender breasts, and other minor maladies. Unless there are particular complications with your pregnancy, such as recurrent bleeding, there is no reason not to have sex during pregnancy—if you wish. If you find that your expanding belly gets in the way, it may be a time to explore the various positions in the *Kama Sutra*.

TRAVEL

Travel is probably more common for women over 35 than for women in their twenties, simply because it often goes with advanced positions at work and with the higher income that usually correlates with more mature age. Air travel is generally safe for women whose pregnancies are uncomplicated, and most airlines allow women to fly up to the 36th week of pregnancy. After that point, the airlines are justifiably nervous about a possible in-flight delivery. If you have any complications, such as a risk of preterm delivery, you should check with your doctor before making any travel plans.

A pregnant woman who is traveling by air should drink plenty of fluids, wear her seat belt at all times, and utilize the exercises provided in the in-flight magazine to avoid pooling of blood in the legs and possible venous thrombosis (blood clot).

Travel to places with altitudes over 8,000 feet can be problematic for women not acclimatized to such heights. This is probably not the time to plan that ski trip to the Rockies. A survey of health care providers at high-altitude tourist destinations indicated that the most frequent problems encountered by pregnant visitors were bleeding complications and preterm labor.

Beyond these cautions, common sense should play a big part in your travel plans. Clearly, if you are close to term or have any complications of pregnancy, you do not want to be far away from appropriate health care.

EXERCISE

Exercise in pregnancy is to be encouraged and there are only a few types of exercise that we will caution against. These are scuba diving, exercises while lying on your back, and probably heavy resistance weightlifting. Recognize that your center of gravity has shifted and that you are at greater risk of losing your balance, so activities such as skiing and horseback riding present an increased risk of falls. Swimming, walking, and using stationary bicycles are excellent ways for the pregnant woman to maintain fitness.

Strenuous aerobics and jogging are good for women who are already habituated to this exercise, and no adverse effects on the pregnancy have been shown in these women. However, pregnancy is probably not a good time to initiate exercise of this sort.

Thirty minutes of exercise daily is recommended, at least five days of the week. When exercising, do drink plenty of fluids and do not become overheated. Because you are burning calories by exercising, be sure to take in enough calories to offset those being used up. If you are not maintaining your proper weight gain, you may need to either exercise less or eat more.

If any of the following symptoms or signs occur while exercising, stop exercising and notify your doctor:

Shortness of breath
Bleeding
Chest pain
Lightheadedness
Headache
Leg pain
Contractions or abdominal cramping
Baby stops moving
Fluid leakage from vagina

WORK

The relationship between working and parenting is discussed in Chapter 2, in the section on considering pregnancy. Now that you are pregnant, this topic is likely to be even more on your mind.

The degree and nature of restriction that pregnancy will place on your ability to work will depend on the type of work you do. As a rule, work that is no more strenuous and exposes you to no more hazards than does ordinary daily life will not pose any threat to a pregnancy. A woman so engaged may continue to work up to her due date, as long as she has no complications of pregnancy. If your work requires strenuous physical work, as in carpentry or farming, you may have to delegate some of the most strenuous chores, if possible; talk with your employer about modifying your work requirements. Even if your job is not physically demanding, you may find that your increased fatigue may make some adjustments necessary. You can't be fired for being pregnant, but your employer's legal obligation extends only to providing you the same short-term disability accommodations that he would give any worker for any health problem.

Whether to work during—and after—pregnancy is a particularly conflict-ridden question for the mother over 35. Many of us are established in successful careers and have reached a good pay and benefits level. Pregnancy provides much cause for introspection on the subject of career.

Here are some of the questions about the interface between work and parenting that you will need to ask yourself:

- Who will care for my child while I work?
- Do I want to continue to work? Full time? Flex time? Is job sharing possible?
- Can I telecommute?
- Who will stay home if our child is sick?
- Who will take the baby for pediatrician appointments?
- Who will prepare our meals? Do the dishes?
- Who will do the shopping?
- What about breastfeeding? Do I want to? How would I manage it during work hours?
- Will there be any time for me . . . just to read a book or watch a TV show?

Many other questions will arise, but the ones above are basic. You would do well to answer them several months before your baby arrives. The answers will be different for each woman.

You may remember Louise and Ted, who were both in their forties when they decided to adopt. Louise, a middle school principal, and Ted, a senior research librarian, resolved some of the questions above by deciding that they would alternate taking leaves of absence from their respective jobs and that Ted would stay home for the first two years of young Owen's life. Since Owen was adopted, breastfeeding was not an issue. Ted was mindful of his need for time out, so they made arrangements to leave Owen with a grandmotherly neighbor for two hours twice weekly.

Michele had decided that for her to handle a rural medical practice and motherhood, she would have to restrict her practice to outpatients only. She opted to breastfeed and took the children to the office with her. After the birth of their second child, when she was 37, her husband stayed home with the children. Sheila, another doctor, restricted her practice to emergency room medicine, where she had the flexibility of working two or three 12-hour shifts per week. She would express breast milk and her husband or the babysitter would give the baby a bottle of it when Sheila was at work. They also supplemented with formula.

Nan, a stockbroker, arranged with her firm that she would primarily telecommute. So did Estelle, a specialist travel agent. Colleen, a diesel mechanic, arranged to job share with a man who was attending college as well as working.

As an older person, you have the experience and maturity to come up with good solutions for yourself. As older mothers and professionals ourselves, we can tell you that no matter what choices you make, you will feel conflicted. Sometimes you will be giving your best to the child and sometimes it will go to the job; rarely will you feel that you have fulfilled both roles ideally. This is one of the most difficult aspects of being a working older mother.

We specifically mention having time to yourself because older parents seem more reluctant than younger ones to leave their precious bundle with a sitter or even a family member. Older parents are often overprotective, probably because in many cases they have waited so long to have the child. Time away from the baby is important to your mental health and to your relationship as partners. All parents have a natural tendency to be parents first and lovers second, but this habit of neglecting ourselves can get out of hand if we do not schedule regular time away from our child. You don't want to wake up at 50 and realize that you no longer remember what you like to do or who you really are, beyond your daily functions as parent and worker. It is easy to bury yourself in the demands of family and work.

A good goal in making lifestyle decisions during pregnancy and later, during childrearing, is to achieve a balance between the various demands on your time and energies and what you need personally for well-being and satisfaction. A baby will give you immense satisfaction and joy, but it is a mistake—for you and for your child—to let him or her become your sole reason for existing. You are a person apart from the child, and this person needs nurturing just as you nurture your baby.

Chapter 15

─────── ∾ ───────

Minor Maladies of Pregnancy

At some point in their pregnancy, most pregnant women experience assorted physical complaints and discomforts. Doctors call these problems "the minor maladies of pregnancy" because they are problematic to experience but have no serious impact on your health or that of your baby. Most of them make their appearance early in pregnancy, and many stay around until the end. Fortunately, not all women have all of them, and there are some simple remedies for some of these maladies. We don't list here that feeling of being like a house on legs; there's not much to be done about it, and it *will* go away.

MORNING SICKNESS

"Morning sickness" is a term that you probably know already. It refers to the nausea and/or vomiting that many women experience in early pregnancy. For most women, this condition improves after they enter the second trimester, but it may persist, return, or occur for the first time at any point during pregnancy. Many women will want to share with you stories of their own morning sickness; for many, it was the first clue that they were pregnant and—now that it has passed—has positive associations for them. We are not sure what causes morning sickness, but we think that it correlates with the rising levels of human choriogonadotrophic hormone (HCG—the basis for your pregnancy test).

If you experience nausea, it is helpful to eat small amounts of food frequently rather than going longer without eating. Somehow, being hungry triggers the nausea as easily as overeating does, so both should be avoided. We advise small complex carbohydrate snacks, like whole grain crackers or fruit, but some women find that lollipops work best. It is often helpful to have something like a dry cracker immediately upon awakening, before you get out of bed. Some women find that various types of tea, for example, chamomile and peppermint, are beneficial, as well as providing fluid and being pleasant tasting. Ginger tea helps many women with nausea. You can make it with raw ginger root or with crystallized ginger. Meals should be balanced, but light. Many women also find that they have unexplainable food cravings and aversions, and it is OK to honor these.

Remedies vary in their effectiveness from one woman to another, but they are worth trying if you are having this difficulty. Acupressure is often helpful; the acupressure wristbands for motion sickness can be used. Acupuncture is not usually recommended during the first trimester of pregnancy, mostly for legal reasons. Vitamin B_6 helps some women and can be taken in small doses (25 mg or less) two or three times daily. There used to be a combination drug available specifically for morning sickness; it contained B_6 and an antihistamine. You can approximate this remedy by taking Benadryl (diphenhydramine) 25 mg, available over the counter, in combination with B_6. The Benadryl is often helpful alone.

Sometimes this minor problem can get out of hand and a woman will develop the problem called hyperemesis gravidarum. In this state, a woman is unable to take any fluids or nutrients without vomiting and she becomes dehydrated and malnourished. This cannot be allowed to continue, because it compromises the well-being of both the mother and the baby, so the woman is usually treated with intravenous fluids and, often, with an antiemetic, a drug to prevent vomiting, most commonly Phenergan (promethazine) or Vistaril (hydroxyzine). If your vomiting is not allowing you to retain any fluids or food, you should notify your doctor. Don't try to assess the situation yourself; you don't feel well enough to be objective.

FATIGUE

An unusual level of fatigue becomes noticeable to most women early in their pregnancy; in fact, for many women this may be the first symptom of pregnancy. While it lasts, this fatigue can leave you with a completely helpless feeling of exhaustion. Michele remembers setting an alarm for 15 minutes whenever she sat down because she simply could not stay awake. Although this problem can be inconvenient, it is not a sign that anything is wrong; it is probably your body's adjustment to its changing physiology. Like morning sickness, the condition usually gets better after about 12 weeks.

Increasing fatigue later in pregnancy can be a symptom of anemia, which is common in pregnancy. Be sure to mention it to your doctor, who will check your hemoglobin and perhaps your blood iron levels. Many pregnant women need supplemental iron.

SLEEP DIFFICULTIES

Several physical conditions of pregnancy can make falling asleep and staying asleep difficult. Especially during the first and last trimester, you may need to urinate very frequently, for the simple reason that the expanding uterus puts pressure on your bladder. Although you empty your bladder just before going to bed, you no sooner fall off to sleep than you awaken with that urge. This is maddening. It helps a little to restrict your fluids in the hour before bed, and lying on your side may help ease the pressure on your bladder. If it's not your bladder troubling you, it may be tender breasts. Some women have very sore breasts in early pregnancy and will awaken if they turn in bed in such a way that some weight is on a breast. Others' breasts are so sensitive that even the weight of a sheet is unbearable. Fortunately, not many women are this badly troubled.

Body aches and itching can both make sleep difficult. If you find that you are achy, a hot bath or strategically placed pillows may alleviate your woes. Warm milk (yes, Grandma was right) can be helpful, and its calcium is good for you. Some pregnant women have a problem with unaccustomed itching of various spots on their body. This is a mostly benign phenomenon, but it can be a low-grade torture for the woman so afflicted. One woman told about lying in bed with her nipples, palms, and soles itching unmercifully. She would fall asleep from sheer exhaustion near dawn each day, about two hours before she needed to arise for work. Delivering the baby cures this symptom, but not much else helps. Mention the problem to your doctor, though, because occasionally itching can indicate serious problems with your liver function that need investigation and may require early delivery of your baby.

Heartburn is another cause of sleep difficulties and is a minor malady all on its own. Obviously, as your uterus expands into your abdomen, there is increased pressure on your stomach, and this can cause you to have reflux of stomach acid up your esophagus. Eat small amounts of food frequently, avoid bending from the waist (what waist, you say?), and sleep with the head of your bed elevated. Be aware of foods that trigger your heartburn and avoid them. You can also take small amounts of antacids, such as Tums or Maalox.

BACKACHE

Given what is happening to a woman's body in pregnancy, it isn't surprising that backache is a problem at some point for most women. During pregnancy, the changing hormones are preparing your body to give birth to a child; this means that your pelvis needs to be able to stretch open, allowing the baby passage through the birth canal. As a result, your pelvis may not be as stable as before you were pregnant; more movement is possible at the various joints. There will be strain on your pelvic ligaments, and this may pull on your lower back and send pain up the back along the shared nerves. Additionally, the growing weight of the baby puts pressure on the pelvis and on the muscles of the abdomen, both of which derive support from the spine. The weight of your breasts, which are larger than you are accustomed to, may give you upper back pain. After the baby is born, you may continue with "mother's backache," which is pretty obviously caused by all the bending over—to pick up, diaper, bathe, and feed an increasingly heavy baby. We know you are happy doing these things for your baby, but it is hard on the back.

Leanne and her husband, Danny, owned a fuel oil franchise. Leanne loved delivering oil but had never much liked the office work. When she was midpregnancy, she began to have a constant upper back ache, and she knew it was from hauling the heavy hoses over her shoulder. She also was so tired that she couldn't stay awake even to eat the dinners that Danny was serving her. After about two weeks of this, Danny put his foot down and insisted that they swap jobs. Their families teased them that impending parenthood was turning them into traditionalists, but staying in the office taking orders and keeping the company's books did make a difference in how Leanne felt. They continued with this arrangement until their son was one year old, at which point, Leanne gratefully returned to the oil deliveries.

To minimize the stresses on your back take some simple precautions. If you are in the habit of bending from the waist, learn the trick of bending from the knees with your back held straight. Ask your family doctor for some hints and exercises to maintain back health. You can also find these exercises online at WebMD. There are very easy exercises that strengthen the abdominal muscles that support the back. Placing a pillow under your knees when you lie down on your back and lying on your side with a pillow between your knees will also help. Positioning yourself this way can rest your back when you are lying down. Get in the habit of daily *gentle* stretching, morning and night, to prevent and ease muscle spasm. Stretch smoothly and slowly, and don't "bounce."

Do not attempt to lift, push, or pull things that are too heavy for you. Ask for help. If you need to do heavy lifting at work, see if some accommodation can be made for you while you are pregnant. Women whose jobs involve strenuous physical activities should explore different ways of doing things during their pregnancies. A consult with a physical therapist or exercise physiologist to learn how best to handle the work demands with your changing body could be very beneficial; it is always better to prevent an injury than have to recover from one. Be aware that your employer has no obligation to treat you differently from any other employee, and if you are unable to perform the tasks involved in your job and alternate work within the company is not available, you may be not be able to continue with that employer. Many different responses to this situation are possible when employees and employers cooperate, however.

Ill-fitting shoes and boots can give you a backache all on their own. Be sure that your footwear is sensible and low-heeled. Such shoes will also make you less likely to twist your ankle or fall.

VARICOSE VEINS

Varicose veins most commonly develop on the calves or thighs and sometimes on the vulva. They look like bluish lumps under the skin and for many women first blossom during pregnancy. Not all women get them; you are more likely to do so if other members of your family have them.

A varicose vein is a dilated vein. In pregnancy, the same hormones that cause the ligaments to relax in your pelvis also relax the connective tissue in the walls of your veins. This change, along with the added weight you are carrying, causes the veins to balloon out. This dilatation will persist after pregnancy, but it may not be as pronounced.

You can minimize and perhaps prevent varicose veins by not standing still for long periods of time. If you have to stand, wiggle your toes or rock up on your toes frequently. This makes the muscles in your legs contract and that squeezes the veins, acting like a pump. Also, do not wear hose with constricting bands at the top; these restrict the blood flow back to your heart and predispose the veins toward ballooning. Sitting with the edge of a hard chair against the back of your knees for long periods can do the same thing.

Do get up and walk around frequently, and elevate your feet at every opportunity. Some women pull out their bottom desk drawer and use it as a footstool. If you can, lie down briefly in the midmorning and midafternoon. This takes the pressure off your pelvic blood vessels.

If you do notice the beginning of varicosities, buy some good maternity support hose—and wear them; they do not help if they stay in your lingerie drawer. (In fact, you can wear support hosiery from the start of pregnancy and perhaps prevent varicose veins.) You should put on support hose first thing in the morning, before the veins start to fill. While you are still lying down, smooth the legs of the hose gradually up over your legs and then pull them the rest of the way either lying or standing. This is best done before rising, but if you need to use the toilet first, return and lie on the bed for at least five minutes before putting on the hose.

CONSTIPATION AND HEMORRHOIDS

Constipation, which many women experience during pregnancy, can be blamed on the hormones of pregnancy and is not serious but can be very uncomfortable. After all, you already feel stuffed. Usually, this symptom can be managed by simple dietary changes and some exercise every day. A nice 30-minute walk every day is good exercise and helps keep the bowels moving too. Make sure that you are drinking enough fluids; you should take in about 2 liters of fluid a day. Eat plenty of fibrous foods, like raw fruits and vegetables, whole grains, seeds, and nuts. If you are just not able to get enough, try adding 2 tablespoons daily of milled flax seed to your cereal or salad. It tastes good, gives you fiber, and as a bonus gives you the good fatty acids that help to keep your skin and hair soft and shining and help you make your own anti-inflammatory substances. There is no down side to flax. If the problem persists and you are distressed, speak to your doctor about a stool softener. *Do not take laxatives.*

Constipation contributes to and exacerbates hemorrhoids, which have been the bane of many a woman's pregnant and postpartum existence. Again, it is the hormones of pregnancy that are the main culprits; they relax everything. The straining to pass stool when you are constipated puts a lot of pressure on the complex of veins around the rectum. Hemorrhoids are basically varicose veins in the anus and rectum. They feel like little balloons at your anus, and they may itch, burn, and bleed. When they bleed, the blood is bright red and is usually on the toilet paper or floating on the water in the toilet bowl. Although the bleeding from hemorrhoids is not in itself serious, you must not ignore any bleeding. Inform your doctor. She or he will undoubtedly have you come in to be checked.

The symptoms of hemorrhoids can be relieved by sitting in a bathtub or basin of warm water, by washing the area with warm water and a soft cloth after defecating, and by using various hemorrhoid suppositories. Prescription suppositories usually have a small amount of a steroid in them. The steroid helps to reduce inflammation and swelling and often gives great relief. An over-the-counter hydrocortisone ointment can also be used. These various treatments are safe to use during pregnancy.

Stretch Marks

Stretch marks, or *striae gravidarum*, distress some women more than others. For women who view them as equivalent to the facial markings of some aboriginal groups, they mark a life passage and may be worn proudly. Other women lament that a bikini will never again look as good. Stretch marks are caused by the overstretching and tearing of the connective tissue fibers as the belly swells with the pregnant (*gravid*) uterus. Some women are more genetically predisposed to stretch marks than others are. While they look violet in color at first, with time stretch marks fade to a silvery white and are much less noticeable; however, they are permanent. Women have tried many remedies to prevent stretch marks, but there is no evidence that any of them works. In our day, women went around smelling like chocolate bars because of all the cocoa butter that we rubbed on our abdomens; today the favored rub seems to be vitamin E oil. These medicaments don't hurt, but it is doubtful whether they help.

PERIPHERAL EDEMA

Swelling of the feet, ankles, and fingers is another common malady of pregnancy. Most women have at least some swelling in their extremities towards the end of pregnancy, and this is part of the huge shift in the hormones and fluids of the body. Many women need to move their rings to their smaller fingers and find that a half size larger shoe is more comfortable during pregnancy. It does help to lie down briefly in the midmorning and midafternoon, drink plenty of water, and get that half-hour of exercise every day. However, these measures may not totally prevent the problem.

If you think that your swelling is excessive or if you have headache, visual changes, or bellyache with it, call your doctor to be sure that something more serious isn't happening. Swelling, although one symptom of preeclampsia, is so common in normal pregnancy that it is no longer regarded as indicative of preeclampsia.

YEAST INFECTION

Yeast infection is a pesky condition that affects millions of women even when they are not pregnant, but it is especially likely during pregnancy. Yeast infections (candida or monilia) of the vagina and vulva cause itching, stinging, burning, pain with sex, and a thick white discharge. The yeast often lives happily in the vagina without causing any symptoms and only becomes evident with pregnancy because the high levels of estrogen that accompany pregnancy encourage growth of the yeast. (Higher estrogen levels in the form of the birth control pills may also stimulate yeast, and you may have experienced this. Also, taking antibiotics, because they diminish the number of healthy bacteria that normally live in the vagina, can predispose one to yeast growth.) Yeast infection is particularly likely in diabetic women, because high blood sugar levels also encourage the growth of the yeast.

Yeast infections are treated with antifungal creams or suppositories, which are safe in pregnancy and can be bought over the counter. This type of infection often recurs. If it persists, see your doctor and have a swab test to check that it really is yeast before trying another course of treatment. Getting your partner to use some treatment as well (cream applied to the penis) can also be helpful; while yeast infection is not regarded as a sexually transmitted disease, it can be passed back and forth between sexual partners.

Finally, we must say that we do not mean to diminish your very real discomfort when we call these "minor maladies"; we have experienced them ourselves and know that they do not feel minor at all!

Chapter 16

———— ❧ ————

Pregnancy Month by Month

This chapter provides a brief overview of what you can expect as the months of pregnancy pass. While this month-by-month calendar describes a normal, uneventful pregnancy, even one complicated by preexisting disease or by conditions developing in the course of the pregnancy will follow approximately this sequence of events. The Resources section of this book lists several excellent general books about pregnancy which provide additional useful information.

Pregnancy is popularly believed to last nine months. In fact, its full duration is 40 weeks. The expected date of delivery is calculated by adding nine months and seven days to the first day of a woman's last menstrual period. Most important points during pregnancy are referred to by week (for example, the week 18 ultrasound). Nevertheless there are definite changes as the months pass—each "month" being somewhere between four and five weeks.

MONTH ONE

During month one, you may not know that you are pregnant. We date pregnancy from the first missed period, because most of the time this is a more reliable marker than trying to pinpoint the date of conception. When you have missed a period and have a positive pregnancy test, we call you four weeks pregnant, although we know that you conceived about two weeks prior to that missed period. This is a convention and gives us a consistent terminology. Home pregnancy tests, if used properly, are very accurate.

By the time you have a positive pregnancy test, your baby, at this stage referred to as an embryo, is implanted in the wall of your uterus. The life journey began when fertilization occurred. Very soon after the sperm met the egg, the resulting cell began to divide—into two cells, then four, then eight, and so on—while the embryo was wafted down the Fallopian tube and into the uterus. There it settled on a hospitable portion of the uterine wall and implanted, usually in the upper part of the uterus.

Almost at once, one part of the embryo began to develop into the baby, one part into the placenta (which provides the baby with oxygen and nutrition and removes waste matter), and one part into the sac that will contain the amniotic fluid that cushions the baby. It is the HCG (human choriogonadotrophic) hormone, produced by the cells that become the placenta, that produce a positive pregnancy test.

During the two weeks between conception and your missed period, the developing embryo is fortunately very resistant to outside influences, such as drugs. This is a good thing, because many women do not yet realize that they are pregnant. If you have been trying to conceive, we hope you have already stopped drinking alcohol and are taking all the healthful steps described in Chapter 1 of this book.

Month Two

In the second month of pregnancy, you may begin to notice these signs:

Your breasts feel tender and larger.
You need to pee frequently, and this need awakens you at night.
You have unusual fatigue and a strange lassitude.
You may feel some lower abdominal discomfort.
You may have morning sickness.

These changes are caused by the increasing hormone levels in your body or the growth of the uterus. As it enlarges, the uterus puts pressure on the bladder and sometimes on the lower bowel. It shifts in the pelvis, and this shift of position can pull on the ligaments, causing the lower abdominal discomfort.

Morning sickness is characterized by nausea and sometimes vomiting and affects half of all pregnant women. It can happen at any time of the day but is most common in the early morning, hence its name. You may develop an aversion to some foods and beverages at this stage. You should avoid all alcohol and go very light on the coffee, tea, and chocolate, consuming no more than the equivalent of about one and a half cups of brewed coffee (see Appendix D for caffeine content of beverages and chocolate). As it happens, alcoholic and caffeinated beverages are high on the list of aversions that some women develop.

The second month is a most important time for organ development in the embryo. At this point, the embryo looks like a tadpole. The heart develops early and is beating visibly by six weeks (this can be seen on ultrasound scans). The brain, face, eyes, ears, stomach, intestines, kidneys, bladder, reproductive organs and limbs are all developing now. The placenta is pouring out large amounts of HCG, and it and the ovaries together are producing estrogen and progesterone. Your blood volume increases dramatically to supply the developing embryo.

During this time and for the remainder of the pregnancy, you must avoid x-rays and unnecessary drugs. Inform *any* health professional by whom you are treated that you are pregnant.

Because you are an older mom-to-be, it is especially important to schedule your first prenatal visit as soon as possible. During this visit, these things will be done:

- Physical examination, including pelvic exam
- Pap smear (if not previously done within the prescribed time interval)

CHOOSING YOUR BIRTHING PLACE

Does this hospital or birthing center offer a range of birthing services?

If I need a Cesarean section, can it be done here? How promptly? (Surgery should be able to begin within 30 minutes.)

If not, how far away is the nearest full-service delivery suite?

Is an anesthesiologist always available? On call (within 20 minutes) or in house?

How far away is the nearest neonatal intensive care center?

Are the rooms comfortable and do they offer enough privacy?

Is the comfort of my support person considered?

Can my baby stay in my room?

When I need to sleep, will the nurses care for my baby for a few hours?

Is there a lactation specialist available to me?

Is my birth method of choice available here?

What is the staff-patient ratio in the labor and delivery suite?

Are childbirth classes offered here?

Are the visiting hours restricted? If so, what are the restrictions?

Is the labor and delivery suite fully staffed or does it depend on "floaters"?

How many of the nurses work only on labor and delivery, and what is their cumulative experience?

- Swabs for chlamydia and gonorrhea
- The panel of prenatal tests will be scheduled
- Ultrasound to confirm dates, heartbeat, and number of embryos
- Prescription of prenatal vitamins with folate, if you are not already taking them

The ultrasound exam will be especially helpful in determining that the pregnancy is indeed in the uterus, not in a Fallopian tube. If you have had a previous ectopic (abnormally located) pregnancy or if you have conceived after a tubal ligation or reversal of sterilization, your chances of having an ectopic pregnancy are increased. Determining how many embryos are in the uterus is important medically and of great interest to parents; multiple pregnancy is more common in older women. Ultrasound will also confirm the age of the pregnancy, so that other prenatal tests can be timed correctly (see Chapter 11).

If you have miscarried a previous pregnancy, you may be reassured by seeing the beating heart of your developing baby on the ultrasound picture.

The second month is a good time to think about where you wish your baby to be born. Depending on where you live, your income, your general health, and your expectations, there may be several options or only one. Where options exist, ask pertinent questions of each hospital or birthing center.

As an older woman, you do face increased risks of problems with your pregnancy. We recommend that you plan to have your baby close to the best possible obstetric and pediatric care available in your area.

Month Three

The fetus is now more than an inch long and your uterus is about the size of an orange. You will not yet have gained much, if any, weight, but you are starting to notice a little roundness just at your waist.

For many women, morning sickness eases off toward the end of this month, but constipation may continue to be a problem and may worsen. The good news is that as the uterus enlarges outward from the pelvis, there may actually be a lessening of pressure on your bladder.

It is around this time that many women begin to have the "bloom" of pregnancy—a glow that resides in the spirit and manifests itself in the face, and makes many pregnant women look radiant.

The famous food cravings of pregnancy begin around this point; you may suddenly develop new passions for particular foods. When she was pregnant with her second child, Michele couldn't get enough baked potatoes. Pickles, strangely enough, are not an uncommon craving. One woman told of craving brown sugar sandwiches! As long as your craving isn't for alcoholic or caffeinated beverages or for foods that would break your budget, there is no harm in indulging it.

If you haven't yet had your first prenatal visit, go now. The examination and tests mentioned in the previous section should be done. It is very likely that your doctor will initiate discussion about testing for Down syndrome, but if not, you should. Even if you have decided that you would not have an abortion under any circumstances, you need to let your doctor know that you have given this thought and have made an informed decision. If you have decided already that you will have a chorionic villus sampling or an amniocentesis, the test will need to scheduled.

Your estimated due date should be well established by now and you can begin to think about booking your childbirth classes and about engaging a doula (described in Chapter 26) or other support people for the birth and the time after.

Many people wait until this time to announce their pregnancy to family and friends, because miscarriage is much less likely after the third month. However, you may want to wait longer to make announcements if you are planning an amniocentesis, as it will give you much significant information. You are not yet beginning to "show" except to those wise women who can read your glow, so you still have time to decide when and how to announce your happy news.

Month Four

Your fetus is now about 6.5 inches long and weighs about 3 ounces. He/she looks like a very tiny baby. And all of a sudden, you feel great! Your energy has returned and you no longer feel limp. For most women, the morning sickness has virtually stopped. And suddenly you are beginning to "show." Your shape is changing by the day; you may literally find that you take off a pair of slacks at night and find them difficult to zip the following morning.

Friends and workmates may know you are pregnant, but you may not want to discuss your plans too widely. Amniocentesis is generally done around 16 weeks, and the results are available in 2 to 3 weeks. Caroline, in her last two pregnancies, waited until after amniocentesis to buy any new maternity clothes, or even to allow herself to think about the pregnancies. She wanted to be sure her test results were normal. Waiting for those test results will be more difficult for a woman who has had children before. They will have recognized the baby's movements from about 14 weeks, whereas first-time mothers don't generally do so until around 18 weeks. "Old hands" also notice other sensations of pregnancy. The pleasurable anticipation is tempered by concern about the health of the fetus and worry that you might have to consider terminating the pregnancy. You will need the loving support of your partner during these weeks.

Month Five

Now your fetus weighs about 10 ounces and is a little over 7 inches long. His skin is covered with a fine soft down called lanugo and he might have a hair or two on his head. You will feel butterflylike movements. On ultrasound, the sex (gender) of the fetus can often be determined at this time. Be sure that you and your partner have discussed whether or not you want to know the sex ahead of birth and that your decision is noted in your records. If you don't wish to know it now, tell the technician who is performing the test. People tend to have strong feelings about this.

Ultrasound technology is extremely sophisticated these days and can give you 3-D photo likenesses of your fetus. In the week 18 ultrasound, besides the sex of the fetus, we can check the brain and face looking for cleft lip and palate, the neck, the heart to see if all four chambers are present, the stomach, kidneys, bladder, and limbs. We can also check the site of the placenta to see if we need to worry about a low-lying placenta.

You will now be having monthly prenatal visits with your doctor or midwife, and your blood pressure, weight, the growth of your uterus, and the baby's heartbeat will be measured each time. The heartbeat is checked with a Doppler machine; the amplification on the machine allows you to hear the heartbeat, too. Some doctors now have their own ultrasound machines. Monthly ultrasounds do allow you to see the growth of your baby, which is nice, but they are not medically necessary.

This is the time to indulge in shopping for maternity clothes or to explore the box of shared clothing that circulates among your family and friends. Try to buy at least one special item of clothing—something that makes you feel beautiful or lifts your spirits when you are feeling large and ungainly.

This is a time to enjoy gestating. You are in between periods of "minor maladies" and you are not yet very large. You may find that your libido has perked up, so this may be a time of very enjoyable sex.

Month Six

By the sixth month, the fetus will weigh more than a pound (500 gm) and be about 12 inches long. On ultrasound, you can see more rounding in his limbs, although he still looks scrawny and wrinkled. The lanugo is plastered down with an ointmentlike substance called vernix caseosa, which is a combination of the output from his little oil glands and his shed epithelial cells. He has eyebrows and eyelashes, and his eyes open and shut.

Around 24 weeks is the earliest that a baby can be born and expected to survive, because "surfactant" is developing in his lungs. Surfactant is a substance that allows the lungs to expand and stay open with breathing. Even so, if he were born now, he would need a premature intensive care nursery. Fortunately, a birth at this age is rare.

The baby's patterns of movement are established now and you can anticipate that he'll be most active when you go to bed at night or get up in the morning or when you do whatever stimulates activity in him.

You will be expanding. You may again be noticing pressure on your bladder, and you may start to be bothered by heartburn, as the expansion of your uterus pushes on your abdominal organs. Your balance may start to feel different; set aside your stiletto heels for the next few months—not least because they will tend to make your back ache. If you start to notice varicose veins or hemorrhoids, take the therapeutic measures described in Chapter 15.

During a monthly prenatal visit at 24 to 28 weeks, you may be scheduled for a glucose tolerance test.

MONTH SEVEN

Now the baby is about 2 pounds and is continuing to grow longer. He can now hear you and the sounds around you. If you have an ultrasound scan around now, you may see him sucking his thumb!

From now until birth, the baby will be gaining weight in fat and muscle, and every week that passes increases his size and his chances of survival if he were to be born early. He is floating still with plenty of room and amniotic fluid; his position in the uterus is not yet a matter of interest medically.

You may perceive your baby's increase in size by its impact on your heartburn and varicose veins and—if you are on your feet too long—backache. (Just remember, these discomforts are usually greatly relieved after you give birth.) If it is winter, you are probably feeling well insulated against the cold. If it is summer, take extra care not to become overheated. You will be extremely tired at the end of a day. All these things are normal.

You are still being seen monthly by your doctor or midwife, and you are gaining weight. At this visit, you may have a blood count to check for anemia and an Rh antibody screen, if this is relevant to you. You should get involved with your childbirth classes now and take a tour of the delivery suite at your hospital or childbirth center. If you haven't already organized your support people for labor and delivery, now is the time to do so.

If you are planning to return to work within six weeks after your baby is born, now is also a good time to arrange for your child care. Having child-care plans in place will free your time after the birth to just rest and enjoy your baby.

Month Eight

By the end of this month, young Einstein will weigh 4 to 5 pounds and will be rapidly gaining weight. He will look nicely rounded and padded with fat and will be very active. Sometimes it will feel like he is having hiccups. He'll respond to your voice and perhaps to music, as well.

You will be starting to feel very stretched and full. The pressure on your stomach and bladder will be increasing and your back will ache more. Your ribs may hurt from the pressure against them. Your shoes may feel a little snug; many women buy "pregnancy shoes" now, ones a half or even a whole size larger than their usual size. Your fingers may be starting to feel a little swollen by the end of the day.

There is less concern about babies born at this stage of gestation. Those born at 32 weeks have a 95 percent chance of survival and a better than 90 percent chance of being free of major health problems. This is good to know, especially if you are carrying a multiple pregnancy, because multiples tend to arrive prematurely.

If you are planning to breastfeed, this is not a bad time to start preparing your nipples by rubbing and pulling them gently several times a day; your doctor may recommend a cream to rub in. You may still get sore nipples, but this preparation is believed to help.

In this month, your baby starts to take up the position he will have when labor starts, usually head first. You will be seeing your doctor or midwife every two weeks now. You have probably been reading a lot of childbirth books all along, but if you have any un-answered questions, ask them now.

MONTH NINE

Now your baby is gaining weight at a rate of a quarter pound at least each week, and his weight more reflects what his size as a new-born will be. He's now about 18 inches long, allowing for individual variations.

From about 36 weeks on, his position in regard to the birth canal will be a matter of great concern. Ideally, he should move into a head-down direction. If he doesn't, you may be tentatively booked for an elective Cesarean delivery. (We describe Cesarean delivery in Chapter 25.) During these last weeks, your doctor may do a limited vaginal exam (disturbing the area as little as possible) to determine whether your cervix has begun to dilate.

You feel progressively more ready to have this birth happen; you

---

PACKING YOUR BAG

Toothbrush

Toothpaste

Hair brush and comb

Nursing bras, if you plan to breastfeed

Cosmetics

Panties — 3 pair

Slippers and/or socks

Nightgown or pajamas — 2

Bathrobe

Outfit for going home

Reading material for amusement

have packed your bag with the personal items that you want with you at the hospital; and you have probably had baby showers and interminable phone calls from concerned friends and relatives. Strangers feel free to pat your pregnant abdomen in the supermarket and ask if it's a boy or a girl. You are visiting the doctor every week and watching the scale register your climbing weight and increasing girth.

Prepare for the birth by pampering yourself. At this point, you may not be sleeping very comfortably and much of you may ache, so do take every opportunity to put your feet up and let your partner take care you. Enjoy luxuriant baths (if you don't feel too awkward to get safely in and out of the tub) or showers—always using a rubber mat in either case. Make an appointment to have your hair trimmed and whatever other maintenance you personally enjoy; you will not have much time and energy for this kind of thing for a while after the birth. Most of all, enjoy "alone" time—it will be scarce in the future.

Chapter 17

———— ∽ ————

Assessment of Fetal Well-being

During even a perfectly normal and unremarkable pregnancy, a number of tests may be done to check on the baby's health. One of the simplest ways of assessing how a baby is doing during a pregnancy is to ask the mother about the baby's movements. Most babies show particular patterns of movement, which become familiar to their mothers. If there is a change in the baby's physical activity, and particularly if movements slow down or stop, your doctor will be prompted to check the baby's well-being by additional methods.

There are several technical ways of checking on the health of a fetus. None is perfect, and many of them tend to overestimate the risk to the baby, that is, they will be accurate for all or most babies who do have a problem, but they will also detect problems in many babies who do not. We say of such tests that they produce a lot of "false positives." Medical interventions based on false positive test results can later turn out to have been unnecessary, though at the time they seemed the reasonable thing to do. Calculating the appropriate response to test results is a process of informed judgment and experience.

CARDIOTOCOGRAPHY (CTG)

Cardiotocography, or CTG, records the baby's heart rate and any uterine contractions happening at the time of the test. It can be used during pregnancy or in labor. Using it routinely on well women has not been shown to improve outcomes. A CTG is generally done in response to particular situations, for example, on women who have raised blood pressure or preeclampsia, on women who have had bleeding (antepartum hemorrhage), on women who have not felt the baby moving, and on women who have gone past their expected date of delivery by more than a few days.

In a CTG, two wide elastic belts are attached around the mother's abdomen, one recording the fetal heart rate and the other uterine contractions. The mother is given a hand-held button to press every time she feels the baby move. The recording is usually continued for 10 to 20 minutes, and a paper printout is obtained. An experienced doctor or midwife can interpret the printout, although there can be differences of interpretation.

On a CTG, we like to see a baseline fetal heart rate of between 110 and 160 beats per minute and a wavy line indicating a continuous variability in the rate at which the heart beats. This means the baby's heart is pumping along, receiving plenty of oxygen. When there is a uterine contraction or when the baby moves, there should be an increase in the heart rate—an acceleration—also a sign of good oxygenation. A perfectly normal baby may have a slower heart rate or a CTG with reduced variability simply because he or she is sleeping. Giving the mother a cold drink or getting her to move around may get the CTG to return to normal. What we don't want to see is any slowing of the heart rate after a contraction of the uterus.

During labor there will, naturally, be contractions, regular or irregular. During late pregnancy there are frequently periods of contractions, which may be felt by the mother, usually painlessly but sometimes with some pain. These practice contractions are called Braxton Hicks contractions, after a nineteenth-century English obstetrician. They vary greatly in intensity and frequency and usually follow no regular pattern.

DOPPLER ULTRASOUND

Doppler ultrasound measures the flow of blood through the baby's umbilical cord. The baby's heart pumps blood out through the cord to the placenta, where the blood receives oxygen and nutrients and gets rid of waste materials. The normal flow of blood is toward the placenta; in the presence of certain problems with the placenta, especially ones associated with high blood pressure in the mother, the umbilical blood flow may slow down, stop, or even reverse. Such changes are a sign that the baby may need to be delivered soon, and they are an accurate indicator of risk to the baby.

Special tests of the blood flow within the baby's heart and brain have been developed, but at the time of writing they are still experimental.

LIQUOR VOLUME

The amniotic fluid, which cushions the baby during pregnancy, is also called the amniotic liquor. It consists of a liquid produced by the amniotic membrane itself (a kind of balloon that completely encloses the baby) and by the baby's urine. At full term, the liquor volume is about 650 to 1,000 cc. The volume of fluid around the baby is a good indicator of the baby's health. There are four "pockets" of fluid, one in each quadrant of the uterus; the pockets are located using ultrasound and their depth is measured. These figures are added together to give an amniotic fluid index—AFI—which is normally between 7 and 20. Higher or lower figures may indicate problems with the pregnancy. Like the umbilical blood flow measurements, AFI is not used routinely in pregnancy but only when a problem is suspected.

MEASUREMENTS OF GROWTH

Under certain circumstances, more detailed ultrasound measurement of the baby's growth is useful: when the mother's blood pressure is raised, which can slow the growth of the baby; when palpation and measurement of the abdomen reveal that the baby doesn't seem as large as would be expected; in the case of twins; when the mother has diabetes, which can cause the baby to be unusually large; and in other situations where the baby's growth is of concern.

The biparietal diameter (BPD), basically the distance across the baby's head at a point above and behind the ears, is a measurement commonly made, together with the circumference of the head and the abdomen and the length of the femur, the thigh bone. Growth is usually recorded on a chart so that progress can be easily noted.

ESTIMATED FETAL WEIGHT

There are various methods for estimating the weight of a baby. And the estimate is just that—not very accurate. It would be different if babies were cube-shaped, but they have arms, legs, heads, and stomachs of varying sizes. Large babies in particular tend to have their weight overestimated. Estimating fetal weight is a bit more accurate than estimating the number of jelly beans in a jar, but only a bit.

THE BIOPHYSICAL PROFILE

From a variety of ultrasound measurements and observations, including the baby's breathing and general movements, a composite statistical profile of the baby's physical condition can be assembled. The process requires an experienced sonographer and is not routinely used, but it can be useful in assessing a pregnancy considered to be at risk.

Chapter 18

———— ❧ ————

Problems That May Arise during Pregnancy

In this chapter we will deal with potentially more serious complications of pregnancy which are more common in older women. It is important to keep this information in perspective—most women have a normal, trouble-free pregnancy. Nevertheless, it is good to be well informed about what can happen and how those situations are dealt with in trying to ensure the arrival of a healthy baby to a healthy mother, so that if a problem does arise you are better equipped to deal with it.

HYPERTENSION

As we explain in Chapter 7, hypertension, or high blood pressure, is a common problem in our society, and is more likely to affect people as they age, so older women who become pregnant are more likely to have hypertension at the start of pregnancy. Hypertension may also develop for the first time during pregnancy.

Hypertension during pregnancy is divided into four categories: (1) chronic high blood pressure predating pregnancy, (2) gestational hypertension, or uncomplicated high blood pressure developing in the second half of pregnancy, (3) chronic hypertension complicated by preeclampsia, and (4) preeclampsia, a serious syndrome characterized by high blood pressure and protein in the urine. Women with chronic hypertension have a 25 percent risk of developing preeclampsia during pregnancy.

The strict definition of preeclampsia is hypertension with protein in the urine occurring after midpregnancy. (Eclampsia describes seizures or coma occurring in someone with preeclampsia and no other cause for these symptoms, such as epilepsy.) Preeclampsia can have drastically adverse consequences for both mother and baby. For the baby, it can retard growth, require early delivery, and sometimes cause death. For the mother it poses a significant risk of seizures, stroke, and kidney damage. Most women with preeclampsia have a successful delivery, and neither mother nor baby suffers harm, but the risk is always there. If a woman has high blood pressure without protein in her urine, preeclampsia is still suspected if she develops headache, blurred vision, abdominal pain, low platelet counts, high serum uric acid, or abnormal liver function tests. Usually, the doctor will act on these signals, because the consequence of not acting can be so dire.

We don't know what causes preeclampsia, but we do know that it is characterized by profound physiologic disturbances in the liver, kidneys, blood clotting mechanisms, and vascular system. There can be ischemia (lack of oxygen due to an impaired blood supply) in the mother's brain, kidneys, and liver, and in the placenta. This condition is life threatening to both the mother and the baby. HELLP syndrome (hemolysis [breakdown of red blood cells], elevated liver enzymes, and low platelet count) is a major complication that can occur even in mild preeclampsia.

If you have any signs of preeclampsia, your doctor will moni

FACTORS PREDISPOSING A WOMAN TO PREECLAMPSIA

- *Preexisting high blood pressure*
- *High blood pressure during previous pregnancy*
- *Diabetes*
- *Multiple-birth pregnancy*
- *Collagen disease, such as lupus*
- *Preexisting kidney disease*

tor your hemoglobin and hematocrit, your liver enzymes, and your platelet count.

In Chapter 7, we introduced you to Hope, a 38-year-old woman who for five years had been treated for hypertension. Once Hope became pregnant, her doctor stopped her medication and arranged to check her blood pressure frequently. Dr. Hassan also explained that Hope would be monitored closely for protein in her urine and that an early sonogram would be done as a baseline to monitor the growth of her fetus. Hope also had kidney function tests done to detect any hidden abnormality there.

Dr. Hassan very appropriately ordered the following tests, to serve as a baseline for early detection of preeclampsia:

- A sonogram to accurately establish Hope's dates, in order to better follow growth of the fetus
- Hemoglobin and hematocrit (part of the routine prenatal panel of tests)
- Platelet count (usually included in the complete blood count and so part of the routine prenatal panel)
- Serum creatinine (an indicator of kidney health)
- Serum uric acid (elevation is a symptom of preeclampsia)

For pregnant women whose hypertension is uncomplicated by any of the factors above and whose systolic blood pressure stays below 179 and diastolic stays below 110, the current recommendation is to suspend antihypertension drugs during pregnancy. There is much controversy about this course of action. The question being debated is whether continuing treatment of mild to moderate high blood pressure reduces the incidence and severity of complications, and if so, whether the drugs used increase the danger to the developing baby. It is known that rates of complications and death are increased for those mothers whose blood pressures exceed 180/110 or who have impaired kidney function. Approximately 45 percent of the maternal deaths due to eclampsia are in older women with chronic hypertension, even though most cases of eclampsia—80 percent—occur in younger women.

Hope's initial tests were normal and she was confirmed in her belief that all would go well. She planned to continue her healthy lifestyle and to carefully follow all directions of her doctor, although she still had reservations about stopping her ACE inhibitor, lisinopril, which had controlled her blood pressure so well.

In her 25th week of pregnancy, Hope began to notice swollen ankles—not just a little bit swollen. Also, she had to remove her wedding rings before they embedded themselves in her finger. She knew that doctors no longer assume that swelling in pregnancy is a sign of preeclampsia, but she did take this symptom as an alert to visit Dr. Hassan sooner than planned. At the visit, Hope's blood pressure was elevated more than usual, with a diastolic reading of 112. There was also a trace of protein in her urine. Dr. Hassan told her that she must go home to absolute bed rest and return to be seen again in two days, saying, "And Hope, by absolute bed rest, I mean that you must be lying down all the time. The only time you may get up is to go to the toilet. You eat lying down, you read lying down, and you must accept that this is the best thing that you can do for yourself and your baby." (Dr. Hassan was so adamant because too many women interpret absolute bed rest in quite a liberal fashion, allowing for quick chores and errands.) Dr. Hassan also told Hope that if her blood pressure was not better and her urine free of protein in two days, she would need to be hospitalized.

Two days later, Hope's blood pressure was normal and her urine was free of protein. Dr. Hassan told her that she would continue to need twice weekly visits and would have to remain on bed rest for the remainder of the pregnancy. Sonograms indicated that the baby's growth was normal, and Hope continued to feel optimistic. She was also happy that she was able to stay in touch with work via the Internet and conference calls. So far her urine remained free of protein and her liver and kidney functions were normal, as was her platelet count.

At 30 weeks, Hope's blood pressure started to rise, but a 24-hour collection of urine was normal. An ultrasound indicated that fetal growth might have slowed a bit, but the baby appeared healthy. By now, Hope was quite bored and a little depressed by her daily routine of rest, rest, and more rest.

At 34 weeks, Hope's sonogram showed distinct slowing of the baby's growth, and she was complaining of a headache and tenderness in her upper abdomen. Her blood pressure was 160/110 and she had significant protein in her random urine specimen. Dr. Hassan immediately admitted Hope to the obstetrical unit at the hospital. Blood samples were drawn and analyzed without delay. Hope had elevations of her liver enzymes and her platelets were slightly low. Dr. Hassan explained to Hope and her husband, who was very anxious, that Hope had HELLP syndrome and that the necessary treatment was urgent delivery of their baby. Delivery of the baby is the definitive treatment of preeclampsia, even if the baby is premature. Fortunately, all signs indicated the baby was holding his own very well.

Hope was prepped for a Cesarean section. Because of fears about bleeding around the spinal cord if an epidural or spinal anesthetic was used (her platelet count being low), Hope was given a general anesthetic, but first an intravenous line was started and she was given hydrallazine to stabilize her blood pressure and magnesium sulfate to reduce the risk of convulsions.

Robin was delivered by an uneventful Cesarean section; he weighed 5 pounds, 9 ounces, was lively, and protested loudly his eviction from the nice warm womb.

Robin's growth had been a concern because hypertension, and especially preeclampsia, can impair the blood supply to the placenta, reducing the baby's nourishment and slowing growth. In the most dire scenario, the fetus can die in utero. The following are symptoms that, when present in the mother, may indicate the necessity for immediate delivery of the baby:

Severe headaches or vision changes
Deterioration in liver functions
Deterioration in kidney functions
Platelet count less than 100,000/microliter
Severe abdominal pain, nausea, vomiting
Suspicion of separation of the placenta from the uterine wall

Signs in the baby that would call for immediate delivery are severe or progressive slowing of growth, recurrent unfavorable fetal monitoring results, or a deficiency of amniotic fluid (called oligo-hydramnios).

The woman who has high blood pressure or has had preeclampsia needs also to be monitored very closely *after* delivery, because there continues to be a risk of the seizures of eclampsia. As many as 25 percent of the cases of eclampsia occur after delivery, usually within the first two days.

Diabetes in Pregnancy

Diabetes, which can exist before pregnancy or start during pregnancy, is discussed in detail in Chapter 7. We emphasize again the need for: controlling your blood sugar throughout your pregnancy, monitoring the growth and well-being of your baby, especially towards the end of pregnancy, and being aware of the possible need for induced labor or Cesarean birth.

Antepartum Hemorrhage

Bleeding appearing vaginally may occur at any time in pregnancy but is particularly of concern once a baby is "viable," that is, likely to survive outside the womb. This point is generally taken to be from 24 weeks of pregnancy, but obviously the more mature a baby is the greater the likelihood of survival and normal development as the child grows up. Sometimes small amounts of bleeding occur during pregnancy for which no cause is ever found, but in general there are two main causes for bleeding of any significant degree.

Placenta Previa

In placenta previa, the placenta develops in the lower part of the uterus, below the baby, in effect blocking the baby's access to the outside world. The placenta may lie partially or completely over the cervix. Placenta previa is still a cause of maternal deaths, especially in countries with limited obstetric care.

In about 25 percent of women, the placenta lies low in the womb early in the pregnancy. This is because the lower part of the uterus, the "lower segment," doesn't begin to expand and develop until later in pregnancy. When this expansion begins, most low placentas move up out of the way of the baby. Only about 1 percent of placentas are "previa" at the end of pregnancy. Sometimes, if the "degree of previa" is very small and the placenta lies to one side of the baby, normal labor can occur because the baby can slip past the placenta and through the birth canal. Where this is not the case, Cesarean section is the safe mode of delivery.

In the vast majority of women with placenta previa, the diagnosis is made by ultrasound before any bleeding has occurred. Then, as the lower segment starts to expand, from about 24 weeks onwards, some of the placenta detaches from the wall of the uterus, causing bleeding but usually no pain. In most cases, this bleeding settles with bed rest, and the pregnancy continues. Several small bleeds like this are common and are acceptable, provided mother and baby are in good condition and the baby is growing. If the placenta continues to obstruct the cervix, a date can be set for a planned C-section, usually around 38 weeks of pregnancy.

The big concern with placenta previa is a sudden large bleed, which would threaten the lives of both mother and baby. And if the mother dies, the baby also dies. Although it is possible to wait and watch a woman with placenta previa, this must be done safely. She may need to be hospitalized for several weeks, so she can be near the operating room, the blood bank, and experienced staff. This is particularly the case if the placenta is located right across the cervix and the woman has had several bleeds already. Sometimes, if a woman lives near the hospital and has good support and transportation immediately available, she may be able to stay home, with the understanding that she will take things easy and come immediately to the hospital if she has further bleeding or any signs of labor. (By the way, placenta previa that has caused bleeding is one of the circumstances in which we would advise against sexual intercourse during pregnancy.) If heavy bleeding does occur, it is usually necessary to proceed to C-section immediately, and sometimes this means urgently, with a general anesthetic rather than an epidural, so if you are one of those few diagnosed with the condition, keep an open mind about your birth plans and remember that having a healthy baby, and mother, is the most important thing.

Placental Abruption

When a placenta that is in the normal place, in the upper part of the uterus, becomes detached from the wall of the uterus, it is called placental abruption. This condition causes bleeding from the blood vessels that supply the placenta. It can be associated with high blood pressure in the mother; rarely it is because of some kind of trauma, such as a car accident; but most of the time there is no obvious reason. The amount of bleeding varies, from slight bleeding that stops on its own, allowing the pregnancy to continue normally, to very severe bleeding, necessitating immediate delivery if the baby is to survive. Severe bleeding is frequently accompanied by pain. If delivery is indicated, it may be possible to induce labor by rupturing the membranes, but often C-section will be needed because distress of the fetus commonly accompanies any degree of placental abruption.

PREMATURE LABOR

Labor between 24 and 37 weeks of pregnancy is called premature or preterm labor (PTL). Prior to 24 weeks it would be considered spontaneous abortion, because the fetus would not be viable. In some places, babies born as early as 20 weeks are counted as viable in birth statistics, but apart from a few miraculous exceptions, fetal survival is not possible before 24 weeks. About 7 percent of all babies (born to mothers of all ages) are born before 37 weeks, 2 percent before 32 weeks. PTL occurs more often in older mothers because they are more likely to be carrying twins (or triplets) and because it is more common when conception has been technologically assisted. Early delivery may also be needed in older women because of raised blood pressure or other age-associated problems in pregnancy.

There are certain specific risks to the baby with early delivery, and obviously the earlier the delivery the greater the risk. Firstly, it is a sad fact that extremely premature babies may die—this is still one of the main causes of mortality soon after birth. The death is often due to difficulties with breathing: the amount of surfactant, which is produced in the lungs of a mature baby and which helps keep the lungs open between breaths, is less than it should be, and the baby develops respiratory distress syndrome. Hemorrhage into the brain can occur and be associated with cerebral palsy and impaired intellectual development. Very small babies are prone to infections, which can be life threatening. They also commonly develop jaundice, which requires treatment.

Having a very premature baby can be one of the most stressful experiences a mother—and father—can undergo. The baby requires constant intensive nursing in a neonatal intensive care unit and is attached to a jumble of wires and beeping devices. Lots of blood tests have to be done; many parts of the baby are bandaged; and usually it is hard to cuddle the baby. Breast milk may need to be pumped or expressed and fed by tube to the baby, and it can be difficult for the mother to keep up her milk supply. There is constant worry about what might go wrong next. Of course, all these things apply to any ill baby who needs to be in intensive care, and particularly to babies who may need urgent surgery soon after birth. But premature babies are so small and helpless that they are particularly challenging emotionally. Today, most premature babies survive and do well. About 90 percent of babies born at 28 weeks of pregnancy now survive and develop normally.

*P*at's son Luke was conceived with assistive reproductive technology when she was 37. Pat had suffered from endometriosis for many years, and she and her husband, Frank, considered her pregnancy a miracle. But the pregnancy was plagued by episodes of bleeding, each one more anxiety producing than the last. Luke just kept on growing in spite of it all, though. At 27 weeks, Pat suffered a severe bleed, an antepartum hemorrhage, and she underwent an urgent C-section with spinal anesthesia. Luke was transferred to the intensive care nursery just steps away from the operating room where he had been delivered, *and for days Pat and Frank sat beside him, watching him as he lay there linked up to a variety of machines. They felt alternately helpless, frantic, and overcome with joy at his presence.*

Luke spent 7 weeks in the nursery. Fortunately, Pat's bleeding episodes had not stressed him, so he didn't have too many problems breathing. He did need treatment for jaundice, and he needed to grow. Finally, when he was at what should have been his 34th week of gestation, he weighed nearly 6 pounds and his parents were able to dress him up and take him home. Luke is now 8 years old, plays baseball with his dad, won't keep his room tidy, and wants to be a vet when he grows up.

Because we have good drugs to help mature the baby's lungs—corticosteroids—and because these drugs take at least 24 hours to work, it is common to try to stop PTL for at least that amount of time, to allow steroids to be given in advance of delivery. The steroids are given to the mother, usually as two injections 12 hours apart, and reach the baby through her bloodstream. Various drugs are used to try to stop premature labor. The most common at the time of writing are nifedipine, salbutamol, and terbutaline; practice varies from one region to another. Once the steroids have had time to be effective and if labor seems inevitable, these drugs are stopped. We don't delay delivery if the mother has a fever or is bleeding. We also will act without delay if there is evidence that the baby is in distress or for some other reason needs immediate delivery.

Like Luke, many premature babies are born by C-section, especially if they are not yet 32 weeks old. The principal reasons for choosing this means of delivery are that the baby is lying in an abnormal position, such as breech, that the labor is accompanied by bleeding, and that the baby shows signs of distress when the heart rate is monitored with the cardiotocography (CTG) machine.

If a woman goes into preterm labor, she is usually transferred as quickly as possible to a hospital where there is a nursery properly equipped to care for the baby. It has been shown that babies *born in* hospitals with such nurseries and specialized pediatric care do better than those born elsewhere and transferred after birth. Transfer of the baby to a nursery elsewhere, which can happen if the baby is born before the mother can be transferred, is alarming for a woman who has not foreseen premature delivery when preparing her birth plan. It is done in the best interests of the baby. Such special nurseries generally have supportive counselors and other staff who are experienced at dealing with the parents of these tiny babies and who will be there to help you through your ordeal.

After about 34 weeks, because the baby generally will not have the respiratory problems of smaller babies, premature labor is allowed to continue. Such babies may need a short time in a special care nursery, but usually they can be held and breastfed like larger babies.

BREECH PRESENTATION

In a breech presentation, the baby is positioned with his head up in the uterus and does not turn. This means that the lower half of the baby lies in the lower part of the uterus, and so this will be the part which first arrives in the outside world if labor and a vaginal birth are allowed to proceed. This would be problematic, for the mother and above all for the baby, as we shall explain. For this reason, most breech babies born in developed countries these days arrive by Cesarean section.

The bit of the baby that lies lowest in the uterus may be the bottom alone (fanny first), the legs being stretched full-length alongside the torso. This presentation is most common with first babies and is called "frank breech." Alternatively, in the lowest part of the uterus may sit the bottom plus the legs and feet ("complete breech"). This presentation is more common in women who have had one or more previous children—and women who have breech babies do show some tendency to do so again in subsequent pregnancies. The least common type of breech is the "footling," in which one or both feet come first. This is potentially the most risky type. In frank breech and complete breech, the baby occupies the lower part of the uterus quite snugly, but in a footling breech there is lots of empty space, and if the water breaks during pregnancy or early labor, the umbilical cord may drop down, with disastrous results.

The potential difficulty with a breech birth is simply explained. In head-first labor, as we shall see in the next chapter, the baby's head gradually molds, or changes shape, to fit the mother's birth canal as labor proceeds. If it doesn't fit, this becomes clear over a number of hours and there is time to prepare for a C-section. With a breech baby, labor in the first stage may go quite well, with the woman's cervix dilating fully; she then starts to push the baby out—legs, bottom, belly, chest and arms, all of which are somewhat smaller and softer than the head. However, if the head is just a bit larger than the mother's pelvis can accommodate, it can become stuck at this point. The baby, unable to get oxygen, either suffers permanent damage or dies.

Over the years doctors have tried many ways to estimate the size of the baby's head in relation to the mother's pelvis. Internal examinations, x-rays, ultrasound, and so on have been used in this quest. At present there is still no reliable way to assure a woman that she can safely deliver a breech baby vaginally. This is not to ignore the fact that very many breech babies have been safely born vaginally—they have. It is simply that vaginal breech birth is potentially more dangerous for the baby than is C-section. A very large study, the Term Breech Trial, the results of which were published in the *Lancet* medical journal in 2000, looked at the outcomes for breech babies delivered vaginally compared to those delivered by planned C-section and found that those delivered vaginally were three times as likely to die or be damaged during birth than those born by C-section. In fact the study findings were so decisive that the trial was ended halfway through, so that more babies could have the benefit of Cesarean delivery.

Many babies seem to like the breech position around the middle of pregnancy—about 25 percent are in this position at 28 weeks of pregnancy—but as the weeks pass most turn themselves around so that by 36 weeks only about 3 to 4 percent are breech. This is when we start to talk seriously about method of delivery to a woman—and her partner—in this situation. Making a decision about birth method should occur only after adequate discussion and after all your questions have been answered. Most obstetricians incline strongly towards planned C-section for breech babies, especially in older women having a first baby. Some are prepared to consider an attempt at vaginal birth, although usually only in women who have been pregnant multiple times before and if: ultrasound measurements of the baby suggest he is not too large, the mother's pelvis is adequate according to whatever criteria are being used, and perhaps if the woman has had a previous successful breech birth. However, the decision needs to be discussed very fully with your obstetrician. If C-section is to be done, it is usually scheduled for a little before your due date, to avoid your going into labor early. But don't worry; the C-section can still be done if you go into labor, even in the middle of the night, albeit with a little more urgency than everyone had anticipated. Breech babies can turn themselves around right up until the last minute, so your doctor will always check the baby's position one more time before beginning surgery.

Another procedure you may be offered, at around 37 or 38 weeks of pregnancy, is external cephalic version (ECV), in which the doctor attempts from the outside ("external") to gently turn ("version" means turning) the baby from the breech position to head-first (cephalic) position. This works better when the baby is a complete breech, because the legs are already tucked up, allowing the baby to somersault into position. It is usual to check the baby's heartbeat before and after this procedure with the CTG, because sometimes the umbilical cord can become tangled up, leading to slowing of the heartbeat and the need for an urgent C-section. Another rare complication of ECV is detachment of part of the placenta, causing bleeding and again possibly requiring a C-section. Women who have had a previous C-section are not candidates for ECV, because of the possibility of rupturing the scar on the uterus; neither are women who have already had bleeding in pregnancy or have elevated blood pressure, because that's another factor associated with antepartum hemorrhage. Notwithstanding this long list of exceptions and risks, ECV is an effective way of dealing with a breech presentation, and it works in about 40 percent of the cases in which it is attempted. You will need to carefully consider all these facts before making a decision regarding ECV in your own case. Many older women, especially those pregnant for the first time, feel that they do not want to expose their baby to the risks of ECV, so they opt for a planned C-section.

If you choose not to have an attempt at ECV, or if it does not succeed in turning the baby, or, as can happen, the little critter perversely turns back to breech, then you will need to be well informed about Cesarean section and be ready to go ahead with it. We deal with Cesarean section in detail in Chapter 25.

Chapter 19

❧

Twin Pregnancy

Twin births are more common in older mothers, both naturally conceived and as a result of assisted reproductive technology (ART, discussed in Chapter 6). There are two types of twins.

Identical twins, also known as monozygotic twins, result when a single fertilized egg divides soon after conception. The resulting two people possess all of the same genetic material. The rate of monozygotic or identical twinning is relatively constant throughout the world, at about 3 to 5 per 1,000 births, and this rate is not influenced by either the mother's age or use of ART.

Fraternal, or dizygotic, twins result when two separate sperm fertilize two separate eggs during the same menstrual cycle; these babies just happen to share the uterus while they gestate, and they are delivered on the same date. They are no more similar in appearance or genetic material than any other siblings. Ovulation producing more than one potentially fertile egg can happen randomly in the general population of women, but it does happen more commonly as a woman gets older, because hormone production is less consistent than in younger women. Obviously, production of more than one egg is more common with ART because the ovaries are deliberately stimulated to increase mature egg (oocyte) production. (As we mention in our chapter on ART, it is no longer common to transfer more than two embryos into the uterus, so multiple births of more than twins are less common than in the early years of ART. Also, many ART embryos do not survive to full-term pregnancies, and this further reduces the incidence of twin pregnancies after in vitro fertilization, but it is still higher than in the general population.)

Each fraternal twin has a placenta and a surrounding membrane.

Because of the double placentas, these twins are sometimes called "dichorionic," which simply refers to the two placentas. The world-wide rate of fraternal twins varies from 5 to 50 per 1,000 births; the higher figures are associated with ART.

Monozygotic twins can have separate placentas and membranes if they separate very early. If they separate a bit later (we're talking hours to days), they may each have their own inner membrane but share the outer membrane. If they separate after 8 days, they may share membranes and a single placenta. We will not address mono-zygotic twins in detail, because they are not more common in the older mother. Fraternal twins are.

Diagnosis of twinning is one of the uses of early ultrasound scan-ning, and often it can determine whether twins are mono- or dizy-gotic. Especially after ART, one of the twins may die and be reab-sorbed by the body, and a single baby will be born. Because of this, remain emotionally guarded about an early diagnosis that you have twins. Wait until two beating hearts can be seen on the ultrasound to act on the information. Lean on your partner for support during this emotionally tense waiting period.

Testing for Down syndrome and other chromosomal abnormali-ties by means of blood tests is not particularly useful with dizygotic twins. Each twin, having his own genetic repertoire, has an inde-pendent risk of abnormality; but the presence of two separate blood supplies makes the blood tests ambiguous because of the overlap-ping of the results from the two babies. Fetal nuchal translucency (the ultrasound that measures a layer of fluid in the baby's neck) has proved to be a more useful screening tool when testing twins.

If invasive testing (chorionic villus sampling [CVS] or amnio-centesis) is to be done on twins, each twin of a dizygotic pair must be tested separately. This obviously doubles the risk of miscarrying, which would mean the loss of both babies. Making decisions about this kind of testing of twins is fraught with difficulty and is emo-tionally taxing. The risk of these procedures with identical twins is the same as with a single baby, because only one twin needs to be tested. CVS of fraternal twins is not recommended, because it is too hard to be sure that the samples obtained are from different placentas. It is easier, and therefore both safer and more accurate, to perform amniocentesis, using ultrasound to guide the doctor and ensure that fluid samples are taken from around each baby. Amniocentesis on twins should be done by a specialist, and in fact, twin pregnancies, especially in older mothers, are usually followed in high-risk obstetrics clinics.

It is *extremely* unlikely with dizygotic twins that both babies will be abnormal. If one baby is found to have a serious condition, you then have the heart-wrenching choice of whether to terminate the pregnancy with that baby and allow the other baby to grow and be born normally. This is technically possible in most developed countries and results in a healthy birth of the remaining twin about 90 percent of the time. This is a very complicated decision and one you should somewhat prepare yourself for prior to knowing the test results. You also need to keep in mind that there is a small possibility that something will go wrong during the procedure. The termination is done by injecting potassium into the amniotic fluid surrounding the abnormal twin. This immediately causes the heart to stop. Eventually, the fetus is mostly reabsorbed, leaving only a small mummified remain to be delivered with the healthy twin.

Other abnormalities incompatible with extrauterine life can occur, and, since there are two babies, occurrence is twice as likely as with a single fetus. These conditions are unusual. Among them is anencephaly, which is a failure of the brain to form. Ultrasound can pick up this kind of problem at about 18 weeks. These pregnancies can be allowed to continue with no significant risk to the healthy twin. If such a situation should happen to you, you will need specialized support throughout your pregnancy.

It is common sense that just about every complication of pregnancy occurs more often in a twin pregnancy; after all, it is basically two pregnancies happening in the same place at the same time. The good news is that today, with our modern techniques for diagnosing and treating complications of pregnancy, the outcomes for both twins are now very good. Multiple pregnancy, regardless of number, is considered high-risk pregnancy and should be followed in a high-risk pregnancy clinic or practice. You will need more expert help, advice, and care than can be offered by a midwife in a regular practice.

The "minor maladies of pregnancy" which we discussed in Chapter 15 are sometimes worse—well, twice as bad—in a twin pregnancy. This is undoubtedly hard to live with, but these are not serious conditions, in that they don't adversely affect your health or that of the babies.

Early screening is recommended. The week 18 ultrasound is usually done, and most obstetricians then recommend a series of ultrasounds to follow the development of both babies. The growth of twins tends to slow after about 30 weeks. With fraternal twins, this is a result of overcrowding in the uterus. In the case of identical twins, it may be that one is, in effect, hogging more of the oxygen and nutrients, leading to unequal growth between the twins. If this inequality is marked, which occasionally happens, it is called "twin-transfusion syndrome." Such a pregnancy needs to be observed in a specialized unit and may necessitate very early delivery, to give the deprived twin a chance of survival.

In twin pregnancies there is a small—about 2 to 5 percent—chance that one twin will die in-utero. This is more likely with identical twins. Rest assured that such an event has nothing to do with your eating habits. You do, of course, need to follow a sensible diet and be sure to take your folic acid and calcium and any other supplements prescribed for you, as we discuss elsewhere. Supplemental iron is often needed in a twin pregnancy. While adequate nutrition is important in ordinary pregnancies, it is even more so for a woman carrying twins.

Premature delivery of twins is more common than full-term delivery. Obviously, there is a limit to how much you can stretch a balloon, and that is true of your uterus as well. Two little passengers require more space than a single one does. Over the years, many interventions have been tried to prevent early labor, but none has been shown to make any difference. If you are showing signs of going into early labor before 32 to 34 weeks, you will be admitted to the obstetric unit and given steroids to help mature your babies' lungs prior to their birth. This gives them a much better chance of survival in the event of premature birth.

Placenta previa is also more common in twins, simply because the double placenta takes up more space and is more apt to impinge on the lower part of the uterus. The larger placenta also creates a greater risk of postpartum hemorrhage because of the larger raw area where the placenta has been attached and because of the over-stretching of the uterus. After delivering twins, a woman is likely to need drugs to help the uterus contract, and she is more likely to need a blood transfusion than in a single birth.

All of the other complications of pregnancy that we have discussed (diabetes, preeclampsia, hypertension, etc.) are more common in twin pregnancies, and they are dealt with in the same way as in single pregnancies. These conditions do increase the probability that you will have an earlier than usual induction of labor or surgical delivery, a precaution to decrease the risk of further complications and death for you and the babies.

Cesarean section rates are definitely higher in the delivery of twins, especially of older mothers and first-time mothers. One reason is that these babies may have been conceived through ART and may represent the woman's last chance at childbirth. Mostly, the high rate of C-sections is because of malpresentations and other complications that are more common in twin pregnancies. After all, it is probably asking too much that both babies would line up neatly with their heads pointed toward the exit. It's just safer in many cases to deliver the babies by Cesarean.

Normal labor and delivery are usually allowed to commence only if the leading twin is presenting head first. Labor proceeds exactly as it does with a single birth. Usually an epidural is put in place, because it is not uncommon for the doctor to need to manipulate the second baby during delivery, and this is definitely uncomfortable if you don't have good analgesia. Soon after the delivery of the first twin, if the second twin is presenting head first, contractions begin again, either naturally or with medicinal stimulation. Soon the second twin will be born, either spontaneously or with the assistance of forceps or suction. Sometimes an experienced doctor will choose to deliver a breech second twin vaginally because the birth canal has just been stretched by the delivery of the first twin, but many obstetricians today would prefer to perform a planned Cesarean section (to deliver both twins) if either is in breech position. If both twins are breech or lying crossways—"transverse lie"—then a planned Cesarean would usually be done. Obviously this is something your doctor should discuss with you and your partner.

Even when twins are born close to term, they tend to be smaller than single babies and may need special care in the nursery for respiratory difficulties, low blood sugar, and jaundice. These are treatable conditions, and special care nurseries are specifically designed to provide this care. Be sure when selecting your birthing place that you will have access to these specialized services.

You can breastfeed your twins, but know that it will be demanding and that you will need a lot of help. Forget about housework and being hospitable to visitors; if you are breastfeeding twins, you should do nothing but eat, sleep, and feed until you feel strong enough to add other aspects of life back into your day. It is reasonable—and may save your sanity—to complement your breastfeeding with formula feeds. This also enables your partner to be an active participant in feeding the babies. It doesn't make you an incompetent mother!

Many larger birthing centers have special resources for mothers expecting twins; all have provisions for high-risk pregnancies. Ask your doctor about your own choices. There are many twin clubs and resource centers, including online chat rooms. You'll find some of these listed in the Resources section at the back of this book.

Part Four

∾

BIRTH

_____

Chapter 20

—— ❧ ——

The Process of Birth

In the next three chapters we will discuss the processes of ordinary labor and vaginal birth. In Chapter 23 we will describe some of the problems that from time to time arise, particularly with older women.

A handy way of understanding the progress of childbirth divides it into four factors:

The passages
The powers
The passenger
The placenta

We encountered this memory aid in medical school, and we think that it is still a sensible way to approach the topic, because it makes clear that there are several variables and that the process is not static.

THE PASSAGES

The birth canal is the passage through which the baby must travel to get to the outside world. This passage consists of the pelvic bones and the soft tissue structures cradled by them. These soft structures are the lower part of the uterus, the cervix, the vagina, and the perineum, which is the area between the vagina and the rectum. The uterus, an upsidedown pear–shaped organ with a neck—the cervix—and the vagina and the perineum are all centrally located within the bowl-shaped bony pelvis. They are attached to the bones by ligaments and muscles. The most important muscles form a wide sling, called the pelvic floor, across the bowl of the pelvis, and the birth canal pierces this sling. You can feel the action of these muscles if you tighten your vagina and imagine an elevator ascending. These muscles are very important in the second stage of labor, as they help to expel the baby at the actual moment of birth.

The pelvis is shaped like a basin with a narrower pedestal. This shape helps to determine the lie of the baby in the pelvis. The pelvis is formed of several bones whose joints are virtually immobile when you aren't pregnant; in pregnancy, hormones act to relax the connective tissue binding these joints. This relative laxity enables the birth canal to expand and allow the passage of its little traveler; it can also give you back and hip pain.

During labor, the baby's head moves down the birth passage, adjusting itself to the passage as it traverses it, in order to bring the head into correct alignment with the exit of the bony canal. The bones of the baby's skull come to lie over one another, and the shape of the baby's head is gently altered, a process known as molding, which safely ensures that the baby's head arrives intact. In your childbirth education class you are likely to be shown a simplified model of a pelvis and a doll, to demonstrate this passage in three dimensions.

The Powers

The uterus is made of smooth muscle. Smooth muscle is muscle that is not under voluntary control—you can't decide to move it as you can your arms and legs. During pregnancy, your uterus enlarges immensely, and much of this growth is an increase in the amount of muscle, in preparation for labor. When labor is well under way, the uterine muscle contracts rhythmically, its activity orchestrated by a pituitary hormone called oxytocin. When labor is induced, a synthetic version of this hormone is administered to start and maintain the waves of contractions. These waves pass from the top of the uterus to the bottom, essentially squeezing the baby downwards. An effective contraction exerts a significant pressure—around 75 mm Hg within the uterus—and lasts up to about

90 seconds. These contractions are painful (we'll deal with methods of pain relief shortly).

In between contractions, the muscles relax, but each time they do, they don't quite return to their precontraction state. With each contraction the muscle fibers shorten a tiny bit. As labor proceeds, the combination of the force of the contractions together with the shortening of the muscle fibers pushes the baby down into the birth canal.

The relaxation phase allows plenty of oxygen to reach both the muscle and the baby. When labor is induced, careful monitoring of the strength and duration of the contractions is necessary to make sure that there is sufficient relaxation phase.

The contractions work to slowly stretch the lower part of the uterus so that the cervix is pulled upward, just as the mouthpiece of a balloon is taken up into the body of the balloon as it inflates. This is called effacement. As this happens, the cervix opens wider and wider into the vagina until eventually a continuous tunnel is formed. This is when you are said to be "fully dilated." It is through this tunnel that the baby is pushed out into the larger world. This opening of the cervix is the first stage of labor, and it is totally involuntary.

In the second stage of labor, the woman uses voluntary muscles to assist the uterine contractions. These voluntary muscles are the diaphragm, the abdominal muscles, and the muscles of the pelvic floor. These are the muscles that push the baby through the vagina; they are the same muscles used to empty your bladder and bowel. You already have an instinctive knowledge of how to push with them.

THE PASSENGER

The passenger, of course, is the baby. When it's time for labor, the baby's head is usually tucked nicely down, chin to chest, to present the smallest diameter to the birth canal. Several weeks or less before labor, the baby's head snugs down into the pelvis, and the baby is said to have become "engaged." Engagement happens earlier with first babies; it is often a last-minute affair with subsequent babies.

As labor progresses, the baby's head descends into the birth canal, through the pelvis, and rotates so that the back of the head—the occiput—comes around to the front, just under the pubic bone. This happens because of the natural shape of the passage. The baby flexes his head down toward his chest more as he descends. As the baby gets closer to the opening of the vagina, he straightens his neck, which pushes his head through the vaginal opening—the top of the head first and then his little face. In the meantime, Mom is oblivious to his efforts, as she aids him with her strenuous pushing. This is hard work and well deserving of the name labor.

Once the head is born, the shoulders rotate their way through the pelvis; this turns the baby's head 90 degrees, back to its original position. The first shoulder appears quickly under the pubic bone and then is followed by the second. The rest of the baby's body slips out almost immediately after the shoulders. The umbilical cord is clamped and cut. Your baby is born!

The Placenta

After the baby is born, the uterine contractions continue, to help deliver the placenta. This usually happens within a few minutes. Once the placenta is delivered, the muscle fibers of the uterus clamp down on the blood vessels in the wall of the uterus and close them (creating the picturesquely named "living ligatures"), to prevent further blood loss. This process is often assisted with medication. Contractions will continue erratically over the next few days ("after pains") and may be strong enough to require pain killers. They will often be triggered during nursing, because the suckling releases that same oxytocin hormone that causes uterine contractions. This is generally a pleasant sensation, but in the days soon after birth, it may cause pain and increased bleeding. We'll explain this further later.

Chapter 21

— ～ —

The Experience of Birth

How does labor feel? When you first begin wondering if something is going on, you may experience what feels like menstrual cramps or you may feel a rippling sensation in your uterus, mildly uncomfortable but not very painful. You will be quite familiar with these feelings if you have been having Braxton Hicks contractions during your pregnancy, but now they seem to be more frequent. You may also have what is termed "a show"; this is a small expulsion of mucus and blood that happens as the cervix begins to dilate and the mucus plug closing the uterus is released. This can happen a few days before you begin to have contractions. In amount, it will be little more than a staining on your underpants; should it be more than that, you should give your doctor a call.

Your contractions will pick up in strength and frequency and become regular enough to time. This happens more rapidly if you have had a baby before, but it may take several hours before a regular pattern of contractions is established in a first labor. Usually, medical advice is to stay at home until your contractions are about 5 minutes apart. If you have unusual circumstances, such as living a long distance from the hospital, discuss the situation with your doctor ahead of time so that you have a plan about when to go to the hospital. If you go to the hospital, are checked, and then sent back home to wait until labor has progressed further, don't feel embarrassed. You have no reliable way to judge how open your cervix is, and no one will think badly of you for playing it safe. This is a common occurrence.

Some women will begin their labor with a gush of warm fluid down their legs or in their bed. This strange-feeling, painless event is popularly referred to as your waters breaking. The sac of amniotic fluid in which the baby floats has broken open, liberating the fluid. Sometimes the experience may be more of an involuntary drizzle of fluid down your leg. Sometimes you can't tell whether your bladder has leaked or your waters have broken, but your doctor or midwife can tell by passing a speculum into the vagina and looking to see whether fluid is leaking through your cervix. There are a couple of chemical tests to check whether it is amniotic fluid that is leaking, but none of these is completely reliable. You may have been having some contractions before your waters broke or they may begin afterward.

Ana's birth experience is typical of many women having their first baby in later reproductive life.

Ana awakened from a sound sleep with the embarrassing realization that the bed was wet. She couldn't imagine that she had wet the bed, but still she was lying in a pool. She quietly crept out to investigate and realized that liquid was running down her legs and it didn't feel like she was urinating. Time to call the doctor's service, but first she awakened Kenyon. Within half an hour, they were at the hospital and Ana was confirmed in her assessment that her waters had broken. She was also about 60 percent effaced (the cervix had pulled up and thinned out 60 percent of the way) and dilated about 3 to 4 cm. The process had begun.

When you arrive at the birthing suite in the hospital or birthing center near a hospital, you will know what to expect because you will have visited the suite in preparation during your pregnancy. Your contractions, assuming they are regular, will start occurring at a rate of about 3 to 4 in 10 minutes, each lasting 60 to 90 seconds; they start at the top of the uterus and move downwards. The contractions will become stronger and more intense and can be more painful than you may have anticipated. This is particularly true in first labors because first labors tend to last longer than subsequent ones. In addition, in first labor, many women are understandably anxious about the unknown—wondering: How long will this last? How bad will it get? How can I do this without humiliating myself? and other such perfectly normal thoughts. At least in subsequent births you have a good idea of what to expect.

We are certainly sympathetic to the idea of totally "natural" childbirth, using no drugs or medical interventions, and we do view childbirth as a natural event, but we have ourselves experienced the pain of labor and do not encourage women to refuse pain medication when they are suffering. You can still be an active participant in your baby's birth without being in agony. Do keep an open mind about all of the options (which are described in Chapter 22); it is reasonable to have chosen a preferred way of giving birth, but be open to whatever may be dictated by the course of your labor and by Nature herself. We have seen many women embark on labor believing that the pain will be no more than bad menstrual pain and that they will be able to cope using a variety of simple measures. Some of them manage to, but many women find that they do need the help of epidurals and other forms of technology, and no woman should feel in any way that this is some kind of failure on her part.

Ana was tucked in bed in the labor suite, with her relaxation tape playing softly, scented massage oils arrayed by the bed, and Kenyon confidently waiting to rub her back and pace her breathing. Suddenly, she felt like she was having bad period cramps. These were erratic at first but gradually became stronger, lasted longer, and were closer together. The breathing techniques she had learned were helpful at first, but the pains kept getting stronger; and before long, it seemed that Kenyon's pacing encouragement was triggering, not relieving, the pain. She knew this wasn't true, but what difference did that make? It hurt like hell. This was not the "discomfort" about which her childbirth educator had spoken. This was more than she needed to put up with. Kenyon asked the nurse to call the doctor, and pretty soon Ana had an epidural in place and was much more comfortable. Three hours after their arrival at the hospital, they were parents of a beautiful little boy. At that point Ana didn't care that she hadn't had the water birth experience and the Trout Quintet CD they had planned for. She was healthy, their son was healthy, and it had all been an awesome experience.

The contractions intensify as the cervix completely opens and the baby gets ready to begin his descent into the birth canal. This is called the transition time, and it segues into the second stage of labor, in which the baby is pushed down and out into the world.

If your waters haven't broken by now, your doctor or midwife may break them artificially (ARM, artificial rupture of membranes). This is done by a vaginal examination and a nick of the membranes with a forceps, an uncomfortable but not painful procedure that results in a whoosh of warm fluid and often increases the regularity and efficiency of the contractions. The doctor will check to see if the amniotic fluid is clear, which is a sign that the baby is healthy, or whether meconium, the material of a baby's first bowel movement, is present, indicating the need for close observation of the labor.

During your labor, you will be assessed at regular intervals by a nurse or doctor to monitor the progress of your labor. Vaginal exams will be done to measure the degree of dilation of the cervix. The person examining you can also feel some bony landmarks on the inside of your pelvis (the ischial spines, to be precise), by which one can measure how much the baby's head has descended. Throughout labor, your blood pressure and pulse rate and the baby's heart rate will be monitored closely. The dilation of your cervix is recorded on a graphlike chart called a partogram; this allows your nurse and doctor or midwife to quickly check on your progress. If your waters have broken or been broken by ARM but your labor is not progressing efficiently enough, an intravenous drip of Pitocin (sometimes called a Pit drip) may be started. This drug (another is Syntocinon) is a synthetic version of the pituitary hormone oxytocin, which stimulates your contractions and makes them more regular and efficient. It is often used to assist labor. If you do have a Pit drip, your baby's well-being will be monitored even more closely, utilizing a fetal monitor that produces a continuous CTG recording just like the one used to assess the fetus during pregnancy; it also records the labor contractions.

You may be allowed to eat lightly or you may be permitted only clear fluids. There is some difference of opinion on this, so ask your doctor about it during one of your prenatal visits. If there is any reason to think that you might need a Cesarean delivery, you will be kept on IV fluids only. It is helpful to move around as much as you feel able during labor. Your birth partner can be of great assistance here, giving you an arm to lean on during a contraction and, if you do have an IV, pushing the pole. It is hard to hold still during labor, and when you are in bed you probably will be searching for the most comfortable position. Be sure to empty your bladder whenever it feels full. You can be grateful that you are having your baby now. When we were medical students, women were given an enema when they first came on the labor ward, and their pubic hair was shaved close. Now, women are not shaved at the hospital, but some of them arrive with various patterns of decorative shaving. We also see jewelry in places we hadn't dreamed of putting it when we were young women railing against the indignity of shaving. Fashions change, in both personal appearance and medicine!

As you enter the second stage of labor, you become aware of an overwhelming urge to push—much like the urge to evacuate your bowels, but stronger. If you have an epidural in place, this sensation may be masked, or it may be ameliorated by pain medication, like Demerol. As long as the baby's heart rate remains stable, this reduction of sensation on your part is not a problem; nature will take its course, and the contractions will continue, bringing the baby's head into the birth canal. Your attendant—nurse, midwife, or doctor—will be able to feel the contractions by placing a hand on your abdomen and will encourage you to push with the contractions.

Experiment to determine your own most comfortable position for pushing. Many women find some version of squatting is best; others crouch on their hands and knees or sit with their backs against their partner for support, bringing their knees to their chest, and digging their heels into the mattress. Others lie on their side (usually left), supported by pillows or their partner and brace their feet against the bed rail or mattress and drawing their knees up in a fetal position. Whatever works for you is the best for you. You will need to shift position to enable the nurse or doctor to check your baby's heartbeat frequently.

You will find that pushing with each contraction is the hardest work anyone can know. It takes every ounce of your energy and concentration. In order to stay the course, you will need to listen to the directions of your midwife or nurse or doctor and spell yourself by consciously relaxing as fully as possible between contractions.

When you are pushing, direct the thrust of your push toward your bottom. As the baby's head begins to emerge, your midwife or doctor will tell you to pant with short breaths. This allows the baby's head to slowly distend the skin of your vaginal and perineal region so that it flowers open, minimizing the risk that these tender tissues will tear. Even so, tears do sometimes occur, and if there is any sign that you or the baby is in distress, the birth attendant may do an episiotomy, a little cut into the skin and muscle of the perineum, to allow a larger opening, so that the baby can more readily slide out. Doing an episiotomy used to be standard practice, but today we wait until we know it is really needed.

Delivering the head of the baby is the hardest part, but you are not finished once the head is out. The shoulders and then the rest of the body are delivered, and then your baby will be placed on your miraculously flat belly. Now you can see and touch your baby. If you didn't already know the baby's gender, now you will. After you have had a few moments with your baby, he or she will be taken to a warming platform to be examined by the pediatrician and cleaned off.

After the baby is delivered, you will experience another contraction or two and the placenta will be expelled. Your midwife or doctor will probably have massaged the top of your uterus through the abdominal wall to help this happen. You will be given an injection of a drug that helps stimulate the uterine wall muscles to contract in order to prevent excessive bleeding. Depending on your doctor's preference or the hospital's policy, this medication may be given earlier, either with the delivery of the first shoulder or around the time of the delivery of the placenta. Putting the baby to your breast also helps stimulate the uterus to contract, as well as being a natural and joyful thing to do.

Chapter 22

—— ❧ ——

Pain Relief in Labor

We have not pussy-footed around the fact that labor is painful and that analgesia should be available to you if you need and want it. You have already learned much in your childbirth classes (if you haven't yet gone, please don't miss them) about how to make labor manageable, and your doctor or midwife is a great source of information about what kinds of pain relief will be available to you. During labor you will be accompanied by a supportive and loving birth partner. This person is usually your husband or life partner but doesn't have to be. As we indicated earlier, some people are just not able to be supportive in the environment of the labor and delivery suite or any situation involving blood and pain. If your partner is one such person, this is simply a quirk over which he has little control. There will be many other opportunities for him to assist you with the baby, and you will be better served during labor by another loving person, someone who will not need *your* support. This might be your mother, your sister, your best friend, just so long as it is someone you feel confident about. You may decide to hire a professional doula, who is trained to help you during labor and after the baby is born (more about doulas in Chapter 26). Your birth partner will be very important, helping you to pace your breathing, rubbing your back when it aches, and otherwise being there for you.

Early in labor, hot packs can help with back pain and the pain of your contractions. Your birth partner can be very helpful in placing and replacing these. You may also find it soothing to lie in a warm bath, stand under a warm shower or walk the corridor. Distractions, like watching a video or playing cards, can also help in the earlier stages of labor. Later, you will not be able to concentrate on such things. Yoga is helpful; the breathing exercises you learn in child-birth classes are based in yoga practice.

Acupuncture and acupressure can be helpful to some laboring mothers, but not all hospitals will allow the practice of acupuncture, primarily for legal reasons. Certainly, acupressure can be done. Some women find self-hypnosis helpful, but it should be employed only if you have become adept at it through diligent use of tapes and practice well in advance of the event.

Injected pain medications are often used to relieve contraction pain. Demerol (meperidine) is most common, but other drugs are also used. The dosage is carefully judged to give you analgesia but not sedate the baby. Unfortunately, these types of drugs often give you more sedation than you might want or may make you nauseated. If you know that you react in this way to such pain medications, discuss it with your doctor ahead of time. An antiemetic, a medication to combat nausea and vomiting, may be given to you along with the analgesic.

In the United Kingdom and Australia, a mixture of nitrous oxide gas and oxygen (once called laughing gas) is often used for pain relief in labor. The laboring woman holds in place the mask through which the gas comes, and can control the amount of gas she breathes in with each contraction. This method is not widely used in the United States.

Epidurals are used quite commonly today in most countries. An epidural involves the insertion of a thin plastic tube, called a catheter, into the space between the vertebrae of the lower back and the membrane covering the spinal cord. Local analgesics and anesthetics can be injected directly through this catheter, bathing the spinal nerves that receive the pain impulses from your pelvic area.

A useful aspect of epidurals is that once in place, in addition to administration of analgesia during labor, they can be used for anesthesia (medication that completely numbs you to pain) if you should need a forceps or Cesarean delivery, and for the delivery of continuous pain medication after Cesarean surgery. They are also handy to have in place should you need any stitches to repair any tears after birth. Many times, they are set up in such a way that you can control the delivery of medication in response to your need.

The amount of medication during the second stage of labor can often be controlled so that you can feel when to push. (As mentioned in Chapter 21, if your epidural does numb your perception of your contractions, you will need a nurse, midwife, or doctor to direct your pushing.) With an epidural in place, you should still be able to move around fairly freely.

Spinal anesthesia (also called a spinal block), a single injection of numbing medication, will be used only if the need is perceived to be short-lived, for instance, if you are about to deliver but it is found necessary to use forceps or perform a rapid Cesarean section. It is a one-time deal, not a continuous delivery system like the epidural. In spinal anesthesia, a longer, thinner needle is used than for an epidural and the needle is placed in the space inside the membrane surrounding the spinal cord. It is used much less commonly than epidurals.

The advantage of epidurals and of spinal anesthesia is that you are awake and alert for the birth of your baby, and you are not groggy afterwards. Risks of these procedures are:

- It may prove technically difficult or impossible to place the catheter for an epidural. This is more likely to be the case for short or obese women.
- The procedure may cause the mother's blood pressure to drop. This is treated by administering IV fluids and turning her onto one side, which takes the weight of the baby off the large blood vessels returning blood to the heart.
- It may not work. For some reason, the medication does not reach the right spot, or reaches only part of the area, and completely successful pain relief is not achieved.
- During placement of the catheter, there is the risk of nicking a vein and injecting anesthetic directly into the vein. The anesthesiologist or obstetrician doing the epidural is aware of this risk and monitors you closely. This is one of the reasons that having a bleeding disorder or being on medications that cause you to bleed more easily are contraindications for having either epidural or spinal anesthesia or analgesia.
- The nerves to your legs may be damaged. This would lead to transient numbness and strange tingling feelings in your legs

that can last for several weeks. It is most unusual for anything more serious to happen.

- A small proportion of women having one of these procedures will have a "spinal headache" if the needle punctures the membrane surrounding the spinal cord, allowing some spinal fluid to leak into the epidural space. Usually increased fluids, along with the tincture of time, will take care of the headache, but occasionally it may be severe enough or last long enough that the anesthesiologist will do a procedure called a blood patch. This entails drawing some blood from your arm and then injecting it into the place where the membrane was punctured. The blood proceeds to clot there, sealing off the little leak.

If at any time during labor you feel you need an epidural or other form of pain relief, ask for it. Remember, the point of it all is not how your baby gets here; it is having a healthy baby and a healthy mother.

Chapter 23

———— ❧ ————

Problems That May Arise during Labor

Labor is a time of critical importance for the future health of your baby. While labor proceeds without serious complications most of the time, it should be watched over by people who are experienced and competent, capable of recognizing problems if they arise, and able either to deal with those problems themselves or to transfer you rapidly into the care of someone who can do so. You and your doctor will have discussed possible complications and planned for them long before your labor begins, and you will have taken these possibilities into account when you chose your birthing place and your birth attendants.

We believe that *all* pregnant women should have some knowledge of the range of problems that can arise during labor well before labor begins. Where older women are concerned, especially older women having their first—and possibly their only—child, doctors and nurses are probably quicker to offer interventions (induction of labor and Cesarean section in particular), and women and their partners more likely to ask for and accept them. The life and health of the child and the mother are the reasons for these interventions, which we describe in Chapters 24 and 25.

INDUCTION OF LABOR

We've talked about many common conditions—hypertension, diabetes, and so on—that may exist prior to pregnancy or arise during it and that can cause problems. When these problems occur, there may come a point when your obstetrician will say that it's time your baby was born, because, given the problems, the baby is likely to do better out of the womb than in it. Also, for various reasons labor may not be happening, even though the baby is full term. We know that once a pregnancy reaches 42 weeks, the placenta starts to be less efficient at providing the baby with food and oxygen, and there is a small but increasing risk of the baby dying. These are the most common scenarios in which induction of labor is likely to be recommended. Any woman contemplating induction should expect her doctor to describe what will be done, why, when, and where, well before the procedure takes place.

If your cervix is "ripe," which means ready for labor—it is shortening, soft as a ripe peach, perhaps starting to dilate—then induction may be by means of ARM, the artificial rupture of the membranes we have already mentioned. This will usually be followed by an oxytocin drip. The rate of the drip will be balanced against the frequency and strength of your contractions, once they commence, so that contractions like those of normal labor will occur. You will be able to move around, but frequent checks of your baby's wellbeing will be necessary.

If your cervix is not ripe, then medication, usually in the form of vaginal pessaries or gel, will be given over a period of a day or so, to bring about the changes that enable ARM to be performed. The drugs being administered are synthetic forms of prostaglandins, natural substances that alter the consistency of the cervix and cause contractions of the uterus. Exactly what medication will be used depends on where you live and the personal preferences of your doctor. Induction of labor should always be accompanied by close observation of your baby's continued good health, usually by monitoring of the fetal heart rate.

FAILURE TO PROGRESS IN LABOR

It is generally accepted by obstetricians, midwives, and maternity ward nurses that labor, whether it starts naturally or is induced, should progress steadily. Spending days in labor exhausts mother and baby and may compromise the baby's health. The days when this was the norm are long gone. Once you are well established in labor, your cervix should dilate, roughly at the rate of one centimeter per hour, and your baby's head should descend little by little through your pelvis. Your progress will be assessed by regular exams in the course of labor.

Sometimes the process slows down and even stops altogether, events more common in women having their first baby. You will recall the rotation of the baby's head we told you about in Chapter 20: the baby's head turns so that the back of the head (the occiput) rotates from the back or side of the mother's pelvis around to the front, the position in which the baby is normally pushed into the world. Sometimes this rotation process halts and the baby stays in a "posterior" or "transverse" position. This can happen when the cervix is completely open (fully dilated), but it can also occur before the cervix has reached full dilation. If the latter happens, the dilation process often ceases also. Having contractions with the baby in the posterior position can cause very severe back pain in the mother.

The solution is for an experienced obstetrician to assess the situation. Generally some Pitocin or Syntocinon will be used to increase and improve contractions in order to see whether normal labor and birth will proceed. Usually an epidural will be recommended, if one is not already in place. The epidural will enable the woman to cope with the length of the labor and the strength of the contractions and still push when the time comes. If full dilation has already been reached, it may be appropriate to assist delivery of the baby with forceps or the vacuum extractor. Alternatively, a C-section may be recommended, particularly if there is evidence that the baby is tired or becoming distressed.

Each woman is an individual and her labor is a unique experience. Each woman should have her particular situation explained to her, so that she can understand, and hopefully participate in, the decisions that are made to deal with a failure to progress in labor. Remember, the "failure" is not due to anything you have or have not done; it is a natural phenomenon.

Fetal Distress

The term *fetal distress* includes many possible situations, for example, that the baby is acutely short of oxygen and needs rapid delivery. Indications of this situation are marked slowing of the baby's heart rate, as shown on the CTG monitor, and further slowing with each contraction. Babies in dangerous situations often pass meconium (bowel contents) into the fluid around them, which provides another marker of distress. However, a baby may show only slight evidence of being stressed or disturbed by labor; perhaps the CTG printout will be flatter than usual and the heart rate less reactive to contractions or the baby's movements.

Several tests apart from heart rate monitoring exist to assess whether a baby is truly distressed during labor. These include taking a drop of blood from the baby's scalp using a tiny scalpel and special glass pipette or tube and testing the sample for oxygen and lactic acid levels. This is called fetal scalp blood sampling. At the time of writing trials are proceeding with fetal oximeters, devices which are placed close to a baby's scalp or face to measure the oxygen levels in the baby's blood. Fetal oximeters are still in the experimental stage.

If fetal distress is definitely present or strongly suspected, it is a reason to proceed soon to delivery of the baby by whatever means is most appropriate. If you are close to achieving a vaginal birth, some assistance by forceps or vacuum extractor may complete the delivery successfully. If things are less far along, a C-section may be the safest option for your baby. Significant fetal distress creates a situation in which there may be little time for discussion or reflection. The baby needs urgently to be brought into the air-breathing world and given all the help of modern pediatrics. This is why we want you to be well informed about all possibilities and keep an open mind when preparing your birth plans.

In the case of mild fetal distress and slow progression of labor, a C-section may also be the most appropriate choice, but you may have a little more time for discussion. Again, however, being well prepared psychologically and having adequate information are essential. Read all you can about these various possibilities and talk to your doctor about his or her practice well before your due date.

HYPERTENSION AND HEMORRHAGE DURING LABOR

These conditions, described in Chapter 18, may constitute reasons either to induce labor or to perform a C-section. Blood pressure can sometimes rise and the signs of preeclampsia appear so rapidly that delivery needs to be arranged immediately. Vaginal bleeding can occur unexpectedly from placental abruption and may necessitate urgent delivery. However, hypertension and hemorrhage only rarely appear for the first time during labor, so you will probably have had time to discuss delivery options with your doctor in advance of labor.

RETAINED PLACENTA AND POSTPARTUM HEMORRHAGE

Not uncommonly, the placenta may fail to separate and be delivered, as we described in Chapter 20. Often the doctor or nurse will be able to perform an internal exam and deliver the placenta without difficulty, especially if you have an epidural in place. However, it can happen that the placenta does not fully peel off from the wall of the uterus but remains in the womb—a "retained placenta"—and then it needs to be removed under adequate anesthesia in an operating room. This procedure may be accompanied by quite severe postpartum hemorrhage (PPH).

PPH can occur without involvement of the placenta, either because the muscles of the uterus have failed to contract tightly to stop the bleeding or because there are tears or lacerations to the uterus, cervix, or vagina. Another possible reason is that, though most of the placenta has been delivered, a small piece, or perhaps some of the membranes, remains inside, preventing the uterus from closing down tightly.

PPH is a major cause of death in women in underdeveloped countries, who unfortunately lack the good obstetric facilities we enjoy. But it still has the potential to kill women in developed countries. This is one of the reasons we urge you to have birth attendants who are skilled and experienced and to have the birth in surroundings close to a full birth suite, operating room facilities, and a blood bank, just in case you need them.

The treatment of PPH is usually quite simple: make sure the uterus is empty (determined by vaginal exam; abdominal surgery is not needed) and that it is well contracted, and sew up any tears or lacerations that have resulted from the birth. If these things are not done, a woman can bleed to death in a matter of a few hours.

THIRD- AND FOURTH-DEGREE TEARS

It is extremely common for vaginal birth to be accompanied by some tearing of the tissues of the vaginal opening. If only skin is involved, this is called a first-degree tear; if skin and some underlying muscle are torn, this is a second-degree tear. An episiotomy is similar to a second-degree tear in that the cut is in skin and muscle. First- and second-degree tears and episiotomies are easily repaired in the delivery suite, although of course this needs to be done with adequate pain relief.

Sometimes, more severe and extensive tears can occur that involve the sphincter muscle that lies around the anus and behind the vagina. This muscle is essential for continence of feces (stool) and gas. A tear of this sphincter is called a third-degree tear. If the tear extends even farther and damages the mucosal lining of the anal canal and rectum, it is a fourth-degree tear. Fourth-degree tears usually also involve the deep muscles of the pelvic floor to some degree.

Third- and fourth-degree tears are serious conditions that require expert surgical repair and careful management until they are completely healed. If they are not properly repaired—and this means with good anesthesia in place and often in the operating room or in a special area of the birth suite—then fecal incontinence, incontinence of flatus (loss of control over passing gas), and pain and difficulties with sexual intercourse may be the result—clearly very undesirable outcomes. After repair, third- and fourth-degree tears need to be managed, with attention to diet, avoidance of constipation, and adequate pain relief, until they are completely healed. Should you experience one of these tears, you would also expect to be checked after some weeks or months and to be asked if normal sexual functioning has returned. And if you have another pregnancy following such a tear and its successful repair, you may want to consider C-section, to avoid a similar problem on the second occasion. Discuss this with your doctor.

Chapter 24

———— ❧ ————

Operative Vaginal Delivery

We briefly mentioned forceps delivery and vacuum extraction when talking about problems that can arise during labor. Both of these instruments are more often used in the birth of babies of older women. More than younger women, they are prone to slower labor and such complications as hypertension during labor. So, what exactly are these instruments?

OBSTETRIC FORCEPS

Forceps are a metal instrument rather like salad tongs that fit snugly on each side of a baby's head within the birth canal and are used to lift the head out as the mother continues to push with the contractions of labor. About 5 percent of babies these days are delivered with the help of forceps.

Forceps have an interesting history. The device was invented by a family of male midwives, the Chamberlens, French Huguenots who emigrated to Britain in the seventeenth century. For more than a hundred years the Chamberlens kept the secret of the forceps to themselves. They would be called to women in obstructed labor, and they would arrive at the patient's house with the forceps in an oak box. The patient's family would be shut out of the bedroom, and the Dr. Chamberlen of the moment would disappear under the bedclothes to perform the delivery—without, it must be said, the help of modern pain relief. Nevertheless, the forceps saved the lives of many women and babies. Fortunately, the secret eventually became public knowledge.

The forceps in use today have been modified to fit safely on a baby's head without damaging the baby, although some marks on the sides of the head and cheeks may be present for a few hours after birth. Adequate pain relief needs to be in place before a forceps delivery is performed, and today that is usually an epidural or spinal. Most forceps deliveries are done because progress is slow in the second stage of labor and the mother is becoming exhausted from pushing, or because the baby is showing signs of distress. The forceps are used when the cervix is fully dilated and the baby's head is well down in the birth canal, with the back of the head—the occiput—towards the mother's front. There is also one form of the instrument, the Kielland's forceps, that can be used to rotate a head which has stayed in the posterior or transverse position, before lifting the head out. It is not uncommon for an episiotomy to be done in conjunction with a forceps delivery, to help deliver the baby safely.

THE VACUUM EXTRACTOR

Used much like the forceps, the vacuum extractor helps deliver a baby when the cervix is fully dilated and the baby's head well down in the mother's pelvis. It is employed for the same kinds of reasons as are forceps—maternal exhaustion, fetal distress, or other problems in either mother or baby or both. A flat plastic or metal cup fits over the back of the baby's skull and a vacuum is created

---

REASONS FOR FORCEPS OR VACUUM EXTRACTOR DELIVERY

- *Fetal distress*
- *Failure of progress in second stage of labor (cervix fully dilated)*
- *Premature birth, to protect baby's head with forceps (rarely)*
- *Maternal exhaustion from pushing*
- *Maternal disease, such as raised blood pressure or heart disease, when prolonged pushing not desirable*

between the skull and the cup by removing the intervening air with a pump. This attaches the baby's head firmly to the cup, which is then used to pull out the baby as the mother pushes with contractions. This sounds worse than it really is; the vacuum extractor is a safe instrument that has been widely used for many years. Following birth, the baby has a soft swelling, called a chignon, on his or her head from the cup, but it subsides after a day or so and causes no long-term problems. Of course, like the forceps—and everything else in obstetrics—competence and experience on the part of the operator are essential. Lacerations of the cervix, vagina, and/or perineum can occur with the use of either of these instruments and would require skilled repair.

Chapter 25

———— ❧ ————

Cesarean Section

Numerous studies have shown that deliveries by Cesarean section surgery are more common among older mothers. This subject is so important to women getting pregnant later in their reproductive years that it merits its own chapter. First, we look at why Cesarean sections are more common now: the reasons are not completely clear, nor are they completely medical. We will give you much information about what a C-section is, how it is done, what you will experience if you have a C-section, and what happens afterwards.

REASONS FOR AND FREQUENCY OF C-SECTIONS

Rates of C-sections increase steadily with rise in the age of mothers, as do deliveries assisted with forceps and vacuum extraction. Indeed, a 1999 study demonstrated that operative deliveries—including C-section, forceps, and suction—occurred in 61 percent of births in first-time mothers over 40. In a recent large study in Boston, 43 percent of first babies being born to women over 40 were delivered by Cesarean. Nationally, the C-section rate for any birth to women of any age is around 22 percent. (It hit 26 percent in 2003—the highest yet.) In some cases there are strong medical reasons separate from the woman's age for doctors to be recommending a C-section; in others, age influenced decisions about Cesarean delivery, not only decisions made by the doctor, but also those made by the woman and her partner.

In the Boston study, many of the Cesareans were done before the mother had begun labor. The most common reason was that the mother had had previous surgery for fibroids; the next most frequent reason was malpresentation, that the baby was not lying head down, in the normal birth position. Both of these reasons are understandable. Fibroids, knotty bits of muscle in the wall of the uterus, are more common in older women. They can interfere with getting pregnant and cause other problems that prompt surgical removal. If a woman has had one or more surgeries to remove fibroids, she is usually advised that it will be safer to have a C-section if she should become pregnant, because the area from which the fibroid was removed can rupture during labor. Malpresentation, as we discuss elsewhere, can be a serious birth complication; and, naturally, it occurs more often with twins, and multiple births are more common in older women. Also, older women in whom the baby is situated as a breech are more reluctant than younger women to try having the doctor shift the baby's position by external version; their doctors may be more reluctant, too. Taking chances, no matter how small, often has less appeal for the older mother. So, Cesarean section at term for breech babies—for whom Cesarean birth has been shown to be safer—is an understandable choice.

Older women are also more liable to undergo an emergency Cesarean after labor has begun spontaneously or has been induced, because labor is not progressing or the baby is in distress. In the Boston study, one or the other of these causes accounted for about 30 percent of the C-sections in women who had gone into labor prior to the surgery. The fear of death or damage to the baby, at a time when the mother may be less fertile, inclines both the mothers and their doctors to more quickly consider a Cesarean delivery for these reasons than do younger mothers and their birth attendants.

Medical indications did not entirely account for all the Cesareans performed in the Boston study. The higher anxiety often felt by older mothers is believed by many doctors to communicate itself to the attending physician and to lower the threshold at which the doctor will consider operative delivery. The option is usually accepted by the woman and her partner, who regard it as safer for the baby. In the study, inductions of labor also occurred at a higher rate among older mothers, not always for very clear medical reasons. The outcome in a certain percentage of inductions will be an emergency C-section, because labor will fail to progress.

Most obstetricians now believe that a Cesarean section, either before labor begins or after a few hours in labor, carries a very low risk of serious complications for an otherwise healthy woman. And older mothers these days are generally healthy and well nourished. A planned Cesarean birth for a second child, or even, given appropriate circumstances, a planned attempt at a vaginal birth after previous C-section, is also likely to be relatively low risk. If the outcome of a Cesarean section is a healthy baby and mother, and the woman is satisfied with her decision, we see this as a success.

Adding to the rate of C-sections worldwide is a recent and growing phenomenon of Cesarean section on request. This is more common in Britain, but it is gaining acceptance in the United States and Australia. South America, where this has been the practice for years, began this trend. A number of reasons have been postulated for the growing popularity of C-section on request. A much-publicized study of British women obstetricians found that many of these women doctors would choose Cesarean delivery of their own baby, even if the pregnancy was absolutely normal and there was no medical reason for the procedure. A major reason given was the possibility of pelvic floor damage during vaginal delivery and consequent sexual problems. This is suspected to be why middle-class and wealthy Brazilian women choose C-sections: vaginal muscle tone, and therefore sexual function, is conserved. Various studies have produced conflicting results about the degree of damage to the pelvic floor by the passage of the baby through the birth canal and the incidence of such complications as incontinence of urine and/ or feces after a vaginal birth; the findings vary greatly for operative vaginal births (forceps or vacuum). These research findings keep the debate alive and vigorous. It needs to be said that, although the chances of subsequent pelvic floor weakness are greatly reduced following a Cesarean, they are not completely absent.

Critics of Cesarean on demand have accused the women desiring this of being afraid of pain, a condition now saddled with the name "tocophobia," fear of childbirth, or of being, as some British newspapers have put it, "too posh to push." We think it is quite reasonable to want to minimize pain in childbirth; avoidance of pain is a normal human behavior. No one has ever extolled the virtue of pain in any other human activity, especially not in a medical context. And there is some pain involved with a Cesarean section. Fear of or avoidance of pain is not an adequate sole reason for requesting a C-section, which is major surgery, but it may reasonably be a factor in the decision.

Having a planned C-section appeals to some women for the sense of control it gives them; they know when and where the baby will arrive. They can be sure that their partners and any other important people will be on hand; working women can make reliable plans in regard to maternity leave. These and other factors may be practically and emotionally very important for some women. These women, like all who consider a Cesarean, must realize that it is not a guarantee that all will go well. All childbirth has some potential risk. Furthermore, there is always the possibility that labor will start earlier than anticipated and require a rapid change of plan.

The women who desire a planned C-section represent one end of a spectrum; at the other end are those women who are adamant about avoiding a C-section. For the latter group, understanding why C-section rates are higher for older mothers is useful to recall. The threshold for offering surgical delivery is lower for older women because there are more medical reasons for C-section in the older mother. If none of these medical reasons applies to you and you remain healthy throughout your pregnancy and you start labor spontaneously near your due date, then there is a very good chance that you will deliver vaginally. Nevertheless, we hope you will keep an open mind about Cesarean delivery, because things can go wrong; and in these situations, C-section can be lifesaving for your baby and even for you. Being informed and considering the possibility in advance will reduce your anxiety should you be faced with the decision unexpectedly. Childbirth is not a test of your womanliness, nor is it a competition.

ELECTIVE VERSUS EMERGENCY C-SECTIONS

The stories of Linda and Bernadette, which follow, illustrate many of the points we make about Cesarean section and the reasons for doing it. First, we need to explain the difference between an elective (planned) C-section and an emergency, or nonelective, C-section. Some people think that "elective" and "planned" mean that the surgery is not medically necessary; this is not the case.

An elective C-section is done for a good medical reason, but the reason is known sufficiently ahead of time that the delivery can be planned. The woman has time to get used to the idea, ask all of her questions, discuss it with family and friends, and discuss any preferences she may have about anesthesia and the timing of the C-section. She may even be able to pick a date, within reason.

An emergency C-section is done because some urgent problem has arisen and the only solution is delivering the baby immediately by Cesarean. Problems can arise either in the course of the pregnancy or during labor. The urgency may be acute, or it may be slightly less so, as in the case of failure to progress in labor but with the baby and mother still in good health.

Linda is a woman of almost 40 who had had a 10-year struggle with endometriosis and was delighted to find herself finally pregnant, on a second cycle of ART. She and husband, Lou, had been going through name books and wondering if it would be just too cute to give their son an "L" name also. With all the difficulties they had conceiving, they are quite sure this will be their only child. Because Linda also had surgery for fibroids, a C-section was planned for 38 weeks of pregnancy.

At 34 weeks, on the day before her routine check-up, Linda awakened with a bit of a headache. She called Dr. Howat's office, and his nurse said to come in right away and have her blood pressure (BP) checked. The BP was up a little bit, and the nurse had Linda lie down in a quiet room while a cardiotocography (CTG) was performed. After her rest, Linda's BP was normal. Dr. Howat read the CTG as also being normal. Just to be on the safe side, though, he ordered some blood tests and asked Linda to do a 12-hour collection of her urine and bring it in when she came for her scheduled appointment the next day. He also commented that the baby was still in a breech position. The next day, Linda's BP was borderline high, but on the normal side. Her collected urine was OK, free of protein.

Two days later, Linda was seen again, and this time her blood pressure was definitely up and didn't go down after half an hour of rest in the office. She was admitted to the maternity floor for close monitoring. By the following day, it was clear that Linda had developed preeclampsia: her blood pressure was elevated even more, and she had significant protein in her urine, demonstrating that her kidneys were not functioning in their normal way. Blood tests showed that her liver was beginning to be affected also.

Dr. Howat sat down with Linda and Lou and told them gently but firmly that the baby had to come out, that the preeclampsia would not improve until the baby was delivered. If allowed to continue, it would compromise the baby's growth and could threaten the life of both Linda and the baby. He recommended a quick delivery and, since the baby was still a few weeks early and not in a favorable position for a safe labor and vaginal delivery, suggested a C-section for a little later the same day.

Lou and Linda were not happy with how things were going but were relieved that a cure for the present problem and a happy ending were in sight. They agreed to a Cesarean delivery with epidural anesthesia, to be done about one hour later. They knew that the pediatrician they'd chosen for baby Layton—yes, why not?—would be on hand and the delivery would be well monitored.

In Linda's case, a C-section had been planned already, because of previous fibroid surgery and the breech position of the baby. As things transpired, the development of preeclampsia made delivery of the baby urgent, and although there was a reasonably comfortable time margin for Dr. Howat to plan the surgery, Linda no longer had the luxury of long-term planning. Bernadette, on the other hand, never anticipated that she might need a C-section.

Aside from a little anemia, for which she'd been taking extra iron, Bernadette's pregnancy, her seventh, had been pretty uneventful. She had often joked that she was born to breed. The biggest challenge so far had been the response of their 12- and 15-year-old daughters, who found it exquisitely embarrassing that their mother was pregnant at the age of 47: "It means they're still doing it. And they're old!"

At the 34th-week checkup, Dr. McKenna noted that the baby was lying fully stretched across Bernadette's uterus—a transverse lie, not uncommon in women with many children. This situation would make a normal vaginal delivery a dangerous proposition, with a likelihood of life-threatening bleeding once contractions began. An ultrasound confirmed that the placenta was lying high up in the uterus and that the baby girl was stretched out across the uterus, appearing quite at ease. With Bernadette's permission, Dr. McKenna gently turned the baby to head first, but she flipped right back to the position she obviously preferred.

Two weeks later, at 36 weeks, the baby's position was unchanged. Dr. McKenna explained to Bernadette that the force of the contractions might turn the baby into the preferred head-first position, but if the transverse lie persisted during labor, an urgent C-section would be needed. It was obvious that the baby could not come out sideways, and there was a danger that the umbilical cord would fall out through the vagina once the waters broke, a condition called "cord prolapse," crimping the cord and cutting off blood supply to the baby, creating an obstetrical emergency. Because of this possibility, Bernadette was told to come straight to the maternity ward if she had any contractions or other signs of labor. Dr. McKenna went on to explain that if the transverse lie persisted at 38 weeks, they would need to talk about a planned C-section. Yes, all of Bernadette's other babies had been very easy and uneventful deliveries, but this little surprise package was not finished with her surprises.

Bernadette left the office feeling stunned; she had never thought that she might have any problems with her pregnancy. She walked over to the hospital's coffee shop to meet her husband, George, a doctor on staff at the hospital. She was glad they had arranged to meet; she hadn't foreseen that they would have so much to discuss. As she sat down, she suddenly felt a gush of fluid down her legs and realized to her alarm that her waters had broken. George jumped from his seat and, phoning the emergency room on his cell phone, ordered a gurney, "STAT!" In about two minutes, Bernadette was on her way to the labor suite.

When the elevator door opened, Dr. McKenna was waiting and whisked them into an examination room. By this time, Bernadette *was aware of a very strange sensation in her vagina. The labor and delivery nurse already had a Doppler on her belly and they were all relieved to hear the baby's heartbeat, loud and clear. Examining Bernadette, Dr. McKenna reported that the baby's hand had fallen into the vagina when the waters broke. The cord didn't seem to be in urgent danger at the moment, but the baby was still lying sideways. "If she wiggles or you start having contractions, things could shift enough for the cord to fall through," observed the doctor. "I'm sorry you haven't had time to get used to the idea, but I want to get you straight to the OR and deliver this baby by a Cesarean now."*

George knew exactly what Dr. McKenna was saying, and he told Bernadette that they really had to do this; she noted how pale he looked and agreed right away. Somehow, the reality of the situation hadn't hit

MEDICAL REASONS FOR CESAREAN SECTION

Elective	Emergency
Malpresentation (breech, transverse)	*Preeclampsia*
Placenta previa not bleeding acutely	*Failure to progress in labor*
Previous C-section or other surgery on uterus	*Malpresentation after start of labor*
Previous stillbirth or death of baby shortly after birth	*Placenta previa with severe bleeding*
Very large baby	*Fetal distress*
Retarded fetal growth	*Prolapsed umbilical cord*
Certain infections in mother	*Placental abruption (tearing of placenta from uterine wall)*
Complicating conditions in mother (hypertension, diabetes)	*Congenital abnormalities in the baby*
Other maternal illness	

her—it all seemed dreamlike. Dr. McKenna assured them that as long as the baby's heart rate remained stable on the monitor, Bernadette could have a spinal anesthetic. Dr. Walsh, the anesthesiologist, had already arrived and was asking Bernadette a lot of health questions, half of which George was answering for her as the whole entourage made its way to the operating room.

ANESTHESIA

The first necessity in the actual performance of a C-section is that the woman have adequate anesthesia. In Linda's case, an epidural anesthetic, like that used in labor by Ana (see Chapter 21), was used. The medication is administered by means of a very thin plastic tube inserted in the back and through which a mixture of anesthetic drugs is injected. After a few minutes, Linda felt a strange sensation of lightness in her legs and belly; she didn't even feel the ice pack on the mound of her belly. She was very impressed by this. In Bernadette's case, a spinal anesthetic was used. The anesthesiologist asked her to curl up as much as her belly would let her, and then felt along the ridge of her backbone for the space between two of her lower vertebrae. She then injected a little xylocaine into the skin to numb the spot, and passed a very fine needle into the space around the spinal cord. A spinal anesthesia injection goes deeper than an epidural. Once the anesthesiologist was certain about the positioning of the needle, she injected a shot of anesthetic sufficient to numb Bernadette's whole lower half for the duration of the surgery. The entire process took less than 5 minutes.

General anesthesia, putting the mother to sleep, used to be frequent for C-sections; this is what Michele had for her first child. That practice is unusual today. Now, a general anesthetic might be used in an acute emergency if spinal anesthesia is not immediately available or in cases where a lot of bleeding can be expected, such as placenta previa. Some women feel more comfortable with a general anesthetic. If you think you would prefer general anesthesia, discuss the subject with your doctor ahead of time. Provided that a woman is made aware of the risks of general anesthesia, it is reasonable for the anesthesiologist to comply with her wishes, after ascertaining that there are no medical reasons against it.

Laura is a woman expecting her first baby at the age of 41. She has never been a hospital patient in her life; she found having an amniocentesis traumatic; and she has been very anxious about the birth throughout her pregnancy. A small fibroid in the lower part of her uterus is preventing the baby's head from fitting down into her pelvis, so she requires a C-section. Her anxiety level is so high that she and her doctor have agreed that a calm, planned C-section with a general anesthetic will be the best option.

Linda was most pleased to realize that her epidural could be left in for 24 to 36 hours after her C-section, allowing her to control her own postsurgical pain relief. This can't be done with a spinal block, but Bernadette was equally pleased with her intravenous pain medication, also on a pump that she controlled. In Laura's case, while she is still asleep some long-acting local anesthetic will be injected around the incision on her abdomen. After she wakes up, she also will receive intravenous pain medication that she can control herself, after which she can use oral pain medication.

RISKS OF ANESTHESIA

Spinal and Epidural

Headache
Technical difficulty
Drop in blood pressure
Allergic reaction to drug
Infection at injection site
Postoperative urinary
   problems
Damage to spinal nerves

General

Aspiration pneumonia
Slowing of respiration
Drop in blood pressure
Allergic reaction to drugs
Damage to larynx
Postoperative respiratory
   problems

The Surgery

We'll follow Linda and Lou through this procedure.

Lou, dressed in green surgical garb and wearing a paper shower cap, sat at the head of the operating table holding Linda's hand and trying to reassure her, although he was himself shaking like a leaf. He watched as Dr. Howat painted Linda's belly with an iodine-based antiseptic. Next, a paper barrier was put up to shield him and Linda from the sight of the incision being made—Lou was glad about that. Linda reported that she felt some pressure—quite a lot of pressure—on her abdomen and then an uncomfortable pinch, but only for a moment. Next she felt a tugging sensation and asked what it was. "We're just about ready to take the baby out," replied Dr. Howat. Linda later recalled it being a bit like having a tooth pulled but on a larger, more visceral scale. For a brief moment, she felt a little woozy, but then the paper barrier was lowered and she saw Dr. Howat holding a squirming pinkish-gray bundle. "Say hello to Layton, Linda!"

A few minutes later, Layton was snuggling against his mom as his dad watched, relieved. Once again shielded from their view, Dr. Howat was stitching together the layers of Linda's uterine muscle, then the layers of her abdomen, and finally her skin. He told her he was using a combination of staples and sutures, but Linda really didn't care much at that point, because she was so taken with the miracle of a new little person.

Because Layton was a bit premature and small, he was soon taken to the nursery, where he had to spend a few days. Lou was able to stay with him there and later to wheel Linda in to hold his tiny hand. Layton was too small to try suckling at Linda's breast immediately after birth, but had he been a full-term baby, Linda would have been encouraged to feed him while her incision was being stitched up.

Bernadette's experience was very similar.

After it was confirmed that Bernadette's anesthesia was working well, an incision was made low across her abdomen, the so-called bikini cut. About 5 minutes later, Baby Amelia announced her arrival with a loud bellow, which quieted as soon as she was laid in George's arms. The pediatrician on call checked her out and pronounced her fit to linger a bit with her parents in the recovery room before she went to the nursery to be cleaned up and meet her siblings. (And we can report that once her older sisters laid eyes on her, they forgot their previous antipathy to the idea of their mother's pregnancy. It seemed that, with the competition to hold her, Amelia's feet might never touch the ground.)

Risks of Cesarean Section

Cesarean delivery is a surgical procedure, and all surgery carries with it some degree of risk. As you would expect, an elective C-section is less risky than an emergency one: there is more time to plan; it is more likely to take place during ordinary working hours when

---

Steps of Cesarean Section

1. *Skin incision, usually horizontal "bikini cut" (Pfannenstiel incision) but may be vertical*
2. *Extension of incision through fat (everyone has some!), muscle and its coverings, and the peritoneal lining of the abdomen*
3. *Incision to open uterus*
4. *Baby delivered*
5. *Placenta delivered*
6. *Medication given to contract uterus*
7. *Uterus and successive layers in abdomen stitched closed one at a time*
8. *Skin stitched closed*

all experienced personnel are readily available; and the reasons for doing the surgery are less acute. However, today, even an emergency C-section can be quite safe and the risks of serious adverse events small.

Bleeding

Some bleeding is inevitable with C-section, because the uterus, which has an excellent blood supply to help nourish the baby, is being cut open. As they say, you can't make an omelet without breaking some eggs, and you can't cut into a vascular organ (one with a very good blood supply) without some bleeding. The bleeding is quickly stopped by the normal contraction of the uterus after the birth; this contraction is aided by the anesthesiologist, who will administer oxytocin and/or ergonovine. The surgeon will quickly stitch up the wound. Sometimes, heavier bleeding occurs, and it is usually adequately controlled by some extra stitches. Rarely, in about 2 percent of C-sections, a blood transfusion is needed. Postpartum hemorrhage can occur after a C-section just as it can after a vaginal birth.

Bernadette was all stitched and feeling very comfortable in the recovery room, daydreaming about holding the baby, drinking coffee, and having a few days just to loll about in the hospital before returning to refereeing the kids. The nurse checked her blood pressure then peeked under the sheet to check the wound. She paged Dr. McKenna, who appeared immediately. After feeling Bernadette's abdomen and rubbing the top of her uterus to make it contract, she ordered another dose of ergonovine to be given through Bernadette's IV. She explained to Bernadette that women who have had several babies have more fibrous tissue within the muscular walls of the uterus, so the uterus doesn't contract as well as it does in women with fewer children. The much-used uterus often needs some help to contract sufficiently to stop the bleeding.

All obstetricians are aware of this risk in "grand multips," women who have had many full-term births.

Infection

Infection may occur in several locations after a Cesarean. A urinary catheter is usually inserted prior to the C-section, so that the bladder will be kept small and out of the way during the surgery. The catheter remains in place for about a day because it is often difficult to urinate on one's own just after any type of abdominal surgery, especially with an epidural. A catheter can always predispose the urinary tract to infection. The symptoms of a urinary tract infection are low-grade fever, pain when urinating, and perhaps an ache low in your abdomen (a little hard to sort out, as you'll probably notice several kinds of ache in that area).

The surgical wound itself may become infected, either on the outside or deeper in the uterus. Sometimes this is just a minor infection with some redness and swelling at some point on the incision. If the infection is deeper, in the uterus, you will have fever, a discharge containing pus from the incision, and more tenderness even than expected in the pelvis. It is now common practice to give a single dose of antibiotic at the time of the surgery, especially for an emergency C-section.

If signs of infection develop, you can be sure that your doctor will check all the possible sources, take appropriate swabs and urine cultures, and will give you antibiotics to fight the infection.

Damage to Adjacent Organs

Not too far from the uterus are the bladder, large bowel, and some very major blood vessels. Obviously, during a C-section there is a potential for damage to any of these structures. In reality, it happens very rarely, especially if a woman has never had any prior surgery in the area. Of the three organs mentioned, the most likely to be damaged is the bladder, because it normally lies just in front of the uterus. In the rare event that the bladder is injured, it should be repaired immediately by the surgeon. In this case, the catheter will be left in the bladder for up to 10 days, to allow complete healing, but normal bladder function can be expected afterwards. Very rarely, one of the ureters, the tubes leading downward from the kidneys to the bladder, may be injured, because the point where the ureter enters the bladder lies close to the main blood vessels of the uterus. Such damage requires expert attention and the presence of a catheter for a week or more.

Damage to the bowel or to large blood vessels obviously also needs to be repaired immediately, as soon as the baby is born and the uterus is stitched closed.

Deep Venous Thrombosis and Embolism

Because of hormonal changes, a woman's blood is more likely to clot when she is pregnant than when she isn't. This is a normal protective process to help your body prevent major bleeding in the hours just following birth. This clotting tendency of the blood is aggravated by varicose veins and the pressure of the baby's weight on the large veins in the pelvis, causing pooling of blood in the blood vessels in the legs during pregnancy. During labor you are moving around a good deal, but lying still on your back, as you must during a C-section, can contribute to the formation of blood clots in the legs—deep vein thrombosis. If bits of these clots break off and travel in the bloodstream to your lungs, they can block the important blood vessels in the lungs—pulmonary embolism—causing sudden respiratory distress and even death. To prevent this, hospitals supply, and require women having C-sections to wear, those elegant white stockings fondly referred to as TEDS, during the surgery and postoperatively. We encourage you to wear them at home for a while. Various methods are used to compress the calf muscles during surgery, to encourage the pumping of the blood back to the heart and to discourage pooling of the blood in the legs. Both Linda and Bernadette had calf compressors on their legs during their C-sections. These machines rhythmically squeeze the calves, encouraging the return of blood to the heart, so that it doesn't sit in the leg veins and clot. Another device provides electrical stimulation to the calf muscles during surgery, so that they contract regularly and squeeze blood back to the heart. During labor, women in the birth suite are encouraged to walk around; there are many reasons for this, but one is to prevent deep venous thrombosis and pulmonary embolism. Women who are at particularly high risk of these two conditions may be given an injection of a blood-thinning drug at or soon after the time of C-section; this practice has been shown to be safe and effective.

CONSEQUENCES OF C-SECTION

Although damage to the pelvic floor muscles and nerves is much less likely—and if it occurs, much less severe—following a planned Cesarean delivery than following a vaginal birth, C-section does not *completely* protect against pelvic-floor problems. Difficulties with incontinence of urine or feces, or pain with intercourse, can occur. The pressure of the baby's head in the pelvis during pregnancy plays a role. When a C-section is performed during labor, the labor may also contribute to pelvic-floor problems after the birth.

In pregnancies that follow a Cesarean delivery, placenta previa is slightly more likely, and the chance increases a bit with each additional C-section. A woman with no C-sections has about a 1 percent chance of placenta previa; a woman with one C-section has about a 1.5 percent chance of placenta previa in her next pregnancy, two C-sections about 2 percent, and so on. This is likely to be of little consequence to most older women, who probably do not expect to have many more pregnancies. We should add, however, that if you do have a placenta previa following a C-section, there is some chance (still very small) that the placenta will be firmly attached to the lower part of the uterus and not separate at the time of delivery, and that a hysterectomy will be required. This serious condition, called placenta previa accreta, is fortunately rare. Again, it is likely to be of less relevance when an older woman is making a decision about Cesarean delivery.

Some studies have shown higher rates of ectopic pregnancy, miscarriage, and stillbirth in pregnancies following previous C-section births, but these findings have not been convincing and are still being debated. Because C-section results in some scar tissue on the uterus, if you require further surgery at some point in the future, in particular hysterectomy, there is a slightly increased risk of bladder damage at the time of that surgery. The risk of each of these consequences is very small and is unlikely to influence a woman's immediate decision about Cesarean section; nevertheless we feel you should be aware of them.

What about the birth experience for the woman who delivers her much-wanted baby by Cesarean? There are now several studies showing that, regardless of the method of delivery, when women feel well-informed about what will happen, involved in decision making, and, where possible, have continuity of care, they are likely to be satisfied with their birth experience. The least satisfied women are those who had to receive urgent obstetric intervention when they had been planning or anticipating an "intervention-free" birth. As we said in our introduction, it is important to realize that, particularly for older women, birth plans may sometimes be upset by events and immediate expert obstetric help may be required.

Does being delivered by C-section affect the baby? Occasionally the baby may get nicked by a surgical instrument in the course of the delivery, an event most likely if the surgery is being done rapidly for urgent reasons and in the presence of a lot of bleeding. This understandable side effect is remedied by a little plastic bandage on the cut or, if necessary, a few stitches. In general, however, the consequences for the baby are probably good. After all, many C-sections are done in the baby's immediate interest; he or she might not survive otherwise. The baby may need special care afterwards, but this is because of the conditions necessitating the C-section, not the surgery itself. For example, a baby born by Cesarean because he was in breech position and his mother went into premature labor would have the problems all premies have. There is also some quite convincing evidence that our current C-section rates are good for babies. A study of more than half a million babies, done in Ireland, showed that, at current C-section rates, deaths of normally formed babies close to term have declined. The authors of this study made clear that it was not just the C-section but the whole package of modern obstetric and pediatric care that goes with it that contributed to these good results. Obviously, the effects of C-sections on mothers and the risks of the surgery are of great concern, and we should be vigilant about our C-section rates and continue appraising them.

Part Five

❧

AFTER THE BIRTH

_____

Chapter 26

—— ❧ ——

Going Home with Your Baby

Many mothers remember a feeling of tremendous vulnerability when they first went home with their new baby. There is a feeling that the world has slipped a bit on its axis and that, although everything is the same as before, it is all completely different. This seems to be a general reaction, no matter how that baby came to be—by birth, adoption, fostering, or through a surrogate. Somehow, this mite of a human being has altered your perception of the world forever.

Postpartum emotions can be tricky until you have reacclimatized to the hormonal changes that are happening in your body and to the many changes in your life. Your feelings may not be entirely as you imagined. You may find yourself being weepy even when you are not sad, sad for no reason, irritable, or impatient. These feelings are normal and transient, but if they persist beyond about 6 weeks, have a chat with your doctor or a counselor. If you are deeply depressed, are unable to experience the joy of your baby, and are experiencing loss of appetite or difficulty sleeping, or if you are doing little but sleeping, talk with your doctor. You may have postpartum depression.

You will be tired in the first weeks after giving birth. Labor is aptly named; it is very hard work. If you have had a Cesarean delivery, you will also be recovering from major surgery and will have the discomforts of a healing incision (more about that later). In any situation, you will have a newborn who wants to eat every three to four hours, regardless of whether it is day or night. Yes, some babies sleep through the night in the first few weeks, but most don't. Even before pregnancy you might have noticed that you don't have quite the energy level you had when you were 20; being a mother over 35 will really bring this to your attention.

Like other experienced mothers, we strongly advise you to nap when the baby naps. Turn off the ringer on your telephone, put a "Do not disturb" sign on your door, and lie down on the bed or couch with a soft mask or such to block out light. You will awaken if the baby cries. In fact, you will awaken if the baby is too quiet. Master the 10-minute cat nap; they can be very refreshing. Strategically placed cushions and pillows to help your recovering body be comfortable can also help you to relax in a minimum amount of time. Soothing music helps to keep both you and the baby calm and relaxed.

As for housework, this is the time to develop a blind eye or to pass your chores to another member of the household. This may be difficult for you if you have been the household manager, doing everything to your own standard. It is time to let go and rearrange your priorities. You need to conserve your energy.

Rita had always been a meticulous homemaker and expert hostess and was on the partnership track at the engineering firm by which she was employed. She and Steve played doubles tennis every weekend and attended at least one evening meeting each week. When they adopted Ryan, Rita's only concession was to take 2 months maternity leave from work. "I figured that since my body wasn't going through any changes, it would be no problem." However, at the end of 3 weeks of being Ryan's mom while keeping a house that looked like one featured in magazine articles and maintaining their pre-Ryan social calendar, Rita was sitting in the doctor's office. She was draped like limp pasta over the consulting chair and patting at her nose with a wisp of cotton handkerchief. She thought she must have some dreaded disease, because otherwise how could anyone be this tired? She left the office laughing, carrying a prescription that read, "Cluttered, dusty house or cleaning service!"

Taking care of yourself is part of taking care of your baby.

If you had a vaginal birth but with an episiotomy, sitting will be uncomfortable for the first week. Make whatever arrangements are needed to minimize the discomfort. Pillows help. Check with your doctor about creams to use on the stitches; he or she may have a favorite to recommend. Sitz baths are soothing, too.

If you've had a Cesarean birth, you will have some perhaps un-foreseen difficulties. For example, arising from a chair will be not only painful but also very hard to do for the first couple of weeks, until the incision begins to heal and your abdominal muscles regain some tone. Soft chairs are more difficult to get up from than unupholstered chairs. Having something upon which to brace yourself or push off—arms on the chair, a sturdy table at its side—can help you lever yourself to your feet. Until your abdominal muscles heal, it is good to hold a pillow or folded bath towel against your abdomen when you arise from a chair . . . or laugh . . . or sneeze . . . or cough.

You will have been given pain medication to take for the first few days, and you probably won't need it for longer than that. You may find that it dulls your ability to enjoy your baby and family by making you groggy. If you want to stop the medication and use other means to lessen pain, try warm compresses and warm showers. If the stitches or staples in the incision are catching on your panties and pulling, try keeping a piece of silky material inside your underpants. Rubbing vitamin E oil or triple antibiotic ointment on the incision can help to keep it pliable and make it itch less. Speaking of itching, if your pubic area was shaved, rubbing lotion into the stubble can soften it and make it less itchy. The silky material can help here, too.

Your body is not a machine, but like machines, it will not function without fuel. Good nutrition is of paramount importance after childbirth, especially if you are breastfeeding. Many of us respond to stress and fatigue by forgetting to eat or by compulsively eating high-fat, high-sugar, high-salt snacks. Neither approach gives us the nutrients that will help to sustain us through this wonderful, but stressful, time. Nutrient-poor snack foods compound the difficulty by leaving you feeling tired and by making it difficult to lose the weight you gained during your pregnancy.

Satisfy your hunger and your need for high-quality calories with plenty of vegetables and fruits, proteins, and whole grains. You will feel better and will soon find that cravings for sugar and fats have gone away. Don't avoid all fats; include good oil, like olive oil, canola, walnut, and flax, in your diet every day. They supply necessary fatty acids. Nuts and seeds are healthy snacks. Soups that can be drunk or spooned from a mug can be particularly convenient fare. You should continue to be careful about fish if you are breast-feeding, because many of the pollutants will be excreted in breast milk. You may find that the most satisfying way for you to eat in this phase of your motherhood is to graze throughout the day. By all means, do this if it works for you, but make sure that by the end of the day you have meandered through all of the food groups.

We cautioned you against any alcohol while you were pregnant, but after the baby is born, a glass of wine or beer with your meal can be pleasurable and relaxing. Just don't overdo it.

Exercise is important. It helps you to regain lost muscle tone in your abdomen. Exercise is also important to the woman who has become a mother through adoption, surrogacy, or fostering, as it raises overall energy levels and helps to keep bones strong. Go for a walk every day. You can take the baby in a snuggle pack or a stroller; the fresh air and exposure to different surroundings are good for her, too.

Every baby behaves differently, and not all are easy. Some cry a lot, have colic, or seem never to sleep. Some have scary tantrums and hold their breath—a variation of normal behavior that doesn't mean your baby was psychically wounded in utero by something you did or didn't think. If you have an extra-challenging baby, you will be even more tired. You must have respite. Seeking assistance doesn't make you a bad mother. It merely means that you are responding to the situation responsibly by providing a way for you to recharge. Recharging doesn't necessarily mean you have to go out somewhere. You may need help just so that you can take a nap. A doula is a wonderful answer to this problem.

Doulas

A doula is a caregiver for *you*, to enable you to take care of your baby. She (almost all professional doulas are women, although men can perform these functions perfectly well) dedicates her time and efforts to whatever you need to be comfortable and rested for your baby. She will start by helping you through your labor and delivery as a professional support person. A recent survey by the Harris Interactive survey company done for the Maternity Center Association showed that mothers gave doulas the highest marks for support during labor—71 percent compared with 60 percent for a family member.

The doula then helps you when you go home. She is not there to take care of the rest of the family, although it is certainly a good idea to have someone other than you doing that. Think of your doula as a personal server, bringing you drinks and snacks, rubbing lotion wherever lotion needs rubbing, running warm baths, bringing the baby to you as you sit in readiness. She may prepare special and tempting breakfasts or lunches for you, but the family cooking is not in her job description. She may help you bathe the baby, but it won't be her job to do the bathing.

In the first weeks after your baby is born, you will need lots of help, especially if you have had a Cesarean birth and your mobility and activities are limited by pain and weak abdominal muscles. If you can't afford a doula, plan well in advance for adequate, responsible assistance from other sources. Relatives and friends can be a great help, or they can be a nuisance and leave you exhausted. They are not helpful if they require you to organize all of their "helpful" activities and if they expect you to be a good hostess or attentive friend. This is your time to be coddled, and if your friends and family cannot give this to you, hiring professional assistance is worth considering. (You will find addresses in the Resources section of this book.)

THE OTHER PEOPLE IN YOUR LIFE

Relationships need tending when a baby becomes part of your life. There is an initial delirious joy on everyone's part, but without careful tending and complete honesty, negative feelings can creep in to your relationships with your partner, your friends, your parents, other children you may have. You and your partner will both be tired, and this will stretch each person's ability to be understanding of the other's viewpoint. If you are a single mother, you may feel isolated with your baby, and out of sync with your friends. In the household, resentments may build over who is expected to do certain chores and pick up various responsibilities. Because the baby consumes so much of your time and energy, your partner and even your friends may feel that you are shutting them out. Your partner may feel jealous of your special bond with the baby and may want to play a larger role in the baby's care but not know how to say so. Sometimes a partner will view the baby as yours and envision no significant role in childrearing. Good communication about such issues during pregnancy will avoid some misunderstandings and set a precedent of openness. Problems that appear after the baby arrives need to be aired with full honesty, and negotiations for compromises made if necessary.

Aimee was married for the second time at age 38 and had not had a child in her first marriage. She was a nurse with a master's degree in public health who directed an oncology clinic. Her husband, Jon, had a grown son and was not interested in going the fatherhood route again. After a year of marriage, Aimee realized that she really wanted to have a child. They discussed the subject and agreed that they would have one child but that Jon would not be a very involved parent. Aimee felt sad about his choice, but their marriage was solid and Jon was loving and affectionate with their baby son when he arrived, so she felt that they had made an acceptable compromise.

There are probably as many parenting styles and adaptations in relationships as there are people. The important thing is to openly and honestly discuss these issues so that you can live and grow well together.

Sexual intimacy between a couple changes after childbirth. It is virtually inevitable that sexual activity will be of secondary interest to a new mother, at least for a while. Her partner, however, may be very interested in resuming intimacy as soon as the doctor permits it. In humans, the urge for sex is not a personal survival urge, and for you it will be competing with needs that will feel more related to survival, such as sleep, eating, and a few moments of solitary time.

Your estrogen levels will be low in the immediate postpartum time and will continue lower than usual while you breastfeed. Besides reducing your libido, this can make your vaginal skin feel dry, thin, and irritable. Under these circumstances, anything entering the vagina feels too similar to a knife to be pleasurable. This happens after childbirth to women of all ages, but as you approach your menopausal years, your hormones are a bit trickier anyway. If the vaginal tenderness persists, it can be effectively treated with an estrogen cream.

Some women's ability to be aroused is hindered by their fear of waking the baby, and sometimes concern that the baby will be emotionally damaged if he witnesses sex between his parents, even though he won't remember it. The answer to this problem is easy. Put your baby in another room, a nursery if you have space, in his own bed. You can set up a monitoring system that will allow you to hear your baby and be vigilant over him without feeling constantly under surveillance yourself.

Probably the best way to thoroughly enjoy the first few months with your baby is to give yourself over completely to taking care of yourself and your baby. Your circumstances may not permit fulfillment of this ideal, but do everything you can to facilitate it in your prebirth planning and postpartum adaptations. The initial months of your baby's life will rush by so quickly that they will seem like a dream, so make it a pleasant dream.

Chapter 27

——— ❧ ———

Breastfeeding

There is no doubt that breast milk is the absolute best food for your baby. In this, the experts agree with Mother Nature. Also, breastfeeding is one of the most satisfying emotional and sensual experiences that a woman can have. Of course, there are plenty of women who, for a variety of reasons, choose not to breastfeed, and that is why there are numerous high-quality baby formulas. Many women, especially those who want to continue with a challenging and absorbing career after childbirth, find the feeding question vexing and anxiety producing. Let us start by saying that your child will be fed and well nurtured regardless of the means, and you need to be confident that breast versus bottle is not a choice that will scar your child's psyche. Either alone can work well; a little of both may be a good choice.

Breast milk is the natural, custom-made food for the human newborn, and your baby will derive great benefit if that is what is given, even if only for a brief period. Breast milk contains the appropriate proportions of protein, carbohydrate, and fat for the baby's needs and is the best source of these nutrients for the first 6 months. It also contains the specific fatty acids, digestive enzymes, vitamins, and hormones that the baby needs at this time. Protection from some infections is transmitted to the baby through the breast milk. (It can also transmit HIV if the mother is infected.)

Breastfeeding has undeniable benefits for both mother and child. The benefits to you are:

- Easier weight loss
- No bottle preparation
- No expense for bottles or formula

- Snuggling with your baby
- Decreased risk of breast cancer

The benefits to your baby are:

- Decreased frequency of ear infections
- Fewer digestive difficulties
- Less infantile eczema
- Fewer allergies
- Less risk of becoming obese
- Less risk of tooth decay

Breastfeeding is regulated by a physical reflex, so it is not something that you need to take classes in, but the topic will probably be addressed in your childbirth classes. The baby has a rooting instinct that causes him to seek the nipple. You'll see how he'll turn and sort of nuzzle at the nearest part of whoever is holding him. This is rooting. When you are going to feed him, you should hold him comfortably near your breast and stroke his lips with your nipple. This will prompt him to latch on and then the sucking reflex will take over. Remember that he hasn't done this before, so it may take a few tries before he really catches on; but be assured, he will.

If you had a Cesarean birth, positioning the baby may be a little awkward at first. You will need someone to hand the baby to you. Position the baby on a pillow or folded throw that has been placed on your lap so as to protect your incision. Within a couple of weeks, you should be able to pick up the baby yourself and put him to the breast without assistance.

A reality faced by many mothers today, and especially by women established in careers who need to return to work before a baby would ordinarily wean, is the difficulty of combining nursing the baby with working outside of home.

Neida is a lawyer who returned to full-time work 3 weeks after her baby was born. Nevertheless, she feels strongly that her baby should be fed breast milk only, so she takes a breast pump to work with her and every three hours goes to the conference room to pump milk. She then refrigerates the milk and takes it home at the end of the day. The in-home babysitter will feed it to the baby by bottle the next day. At night, Neida enjoys the closeness of suckling little Josh and smelling his fresh baby smell.

Michele's babies, both born when she was over 35 and in the early years of a very busy country practice, were office babies—the nursing baby went to work with her. This enabled Michele to fully breastfeed until the babies were over 6 months old. Of course, not all women have this choice.

Tammy works as an architectural assistant. She was not able to bring her baby to the office. Her solution was to breastfeed in early morning and at night and to provide her babysitter with expressed milk or formula to feed little Kyle while she herself was at work.

Flexibility is the key, as it is to most of the challenges of being an older mom.

You may be advised not to give a breastfeeding baby a bottle early on because the bottle nipple is easier for him to suck and he may get lazy at sucking your nipple. Although this advice is common, most women who have had to use a bottle in the first month have not found it a great difficulty. Often, squeezing a little bead of milk out of the breast so that he can smell and taste it will motivate the baby to latch on.

If you are breastfeeding, you will need to take great care to remain adequately hydrated. Be mindful of this need for fluids and drink them frequently. If you have returned to work, keep a water bottle handy so that you won't forget to drink. You also need to relax (we were taught that nursing mothers should drink a bottle of stout each day, which would help). Your hunger level will probably ensure that you get enough nutrition, but make sure that it is of high quality. We usually suggest that a nursing mother also continue her prenatal vitamins while she is nursing.

Cracked nipples are a painful consequence of breastfeeding but not a reason to stop nursing. You can buy cone-shaped plastic nipple shields or nipple guards, and they will protect you against too-strong sucking by your baby. Applying a gentle lubricating lotion to the nipples at least twice daily also helps tremendously.

Breast infections occasionally occur but are also not usually a reason to stop nursing. Most of these infections are very treatable and often become worse if you suddenly stop nursing, which allows the breast to become engorged.

Two other difficulties you may (or may not) encounter are breast engorgement and inappropriate let down (when your milk releases into the ducts and the nipple but you aren't nursing). Both can be troublesome, especially when you've returned to work. Routine emptying of the breasts will lessen the likelihood of both conditions. Michele recalls her experience with let down the first time she went to a hospital committee meeting after her son was born. She was the only woman on staff. There she was at a round table with several other doctors, discussing an audit of charts, when the front of her sweater became suddenly sodden. She employed the old arms crossed on the chest posture (the pressure helps to stop the flow) and prayed that they hadn't noticed. You probably will have similar experiences, and the best we can suggest is to avoid very light and very dark clothes, as these seem to show the milk stains more than medium tones. Also, putting pressure against the front of the breast does curb the flow, and you may learn to anticipate let down and press before the flow begins.

Obviously, many women choose not to breastfeed. The reasons vary, and no woman needs to justify this decision. You know your circumstances and yourself better than anyone else does. Formula feeding provides scientifically calibrated nutrition and is quite healthy for your baby. It is not the pediatrician-preferred method, but it is sound. Being a mother is not easy at any age, and you need not beat up on yourself for making the choices that seem to make it work best for you.

Bottlefeeding, whether of breast milk or formula, allows you to share the duties and privileges of feeding the baby with other family members and caregivers. It is important that the baby be held when being fed; it maintains the proper angle for the nipple to enter the mouth and helps ensure that the baby receives the holding and closeness that are also necessary for normal development. Besides, it is very nice to hold a baby and to feel his silken skin against your fingers. And when he opens his eyes and you see recognition in them, there is no greater thrill.

Formula feeding used to be a lot of work, but with ready-mixed formula, dishwashers, and disposable bottle liners, things are much easier today. If you mix the formula, it needs to be made up precisely according to the directions given on the container. Babies can get very sick from having the proportion of water to solids wrong. This won't happen if you use premixed formula or are scrupulous in measuring and following mixing directions. Women used to spend a lot of time boiling bottles to ensure sterility; sterility is still necessary, but dishwashers have made it much easier.

Formula feeding may prove a necessary supplement if you have a multiple birth (Can you imagine nursing triplets?), although many women do manage to nurse twins fully. Women who have babies after having had breast cancer may have diminished or no milk supply from the affected breast. Again, excellent formulas are readily available as a supplement or substitute.

For many women, at least some degree of formula feeding is necessary if they are to return to work. Many women do not have the luxury of using a conference room or assigning their own time priorities at work the way Neida and Michele did. Helene's situation is probably more typical.

Helene's pregnancy at age 41 was a huge surprise. She and her husband already had two teenagers just about ready for college. Stopping work — she is in customer service in a large department store — was not an option for Helene if they were to be able to help their children attend college. She felt a bit guilty about not being able to breastfeed Kara, because she had nursed Kit and Kim, but she couldn't afford to stay home with this baby. She nursed little Kara for the 2 weeks of maternity leave that she took. "Then Kara had to go on formula so I could go back to work. My employer is good enough to have day care on site, but they wouldn't let me take a nursing break or even a pumping break."

There are many formulas on the market. Pay no attention to advertising or your girlfriend or your mother-in-law. Your pediatrician will prescribe a formula that is right for your baby's needs, and you should stick with that one unless you and the doctor see a reason to change the formula. Discuss any concerns you may have. Like you, your pediatrician wants what is best for your baby.

Chapter 28

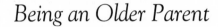

Being an Older Parent

Throughout the ages, no matter what childrearing fashions were in vogue, most children have become well adjusted and responsible citizens. You should keep this well in mind, because as you try to juggle all of your responsibilities and be the best mother that ever was, your self-confidence will erode, and you may be left with little sense of self. If you are kind to yourself and your child and your partner, and apply yourself conscientiously to your job and the myriad other concerns that fill a busy life, one of the legacies you will give your child is the observation and memory of how you balanced your life. This will be more of a lifeline in your child's adulthood than the memory of a cooked breakfast every day would be.

It is interesting to observe older and younger parents and see how they differ. Younger parents seem more relaxed about matters of health and safety, perhaps because they themselves have little sense of mortality yet. Older parents seem more relaxed about certain behaviors, with the result that their children may sometimes be viewed as indulged. Other older parents may be stricter, because they either mimic the code by which they were raised or because they haven't the energy to deal with a chaotic, child-centered household. Older parents usually have more money to spend on their children, and their children are therefore more likely to be enrolled in private, for-payment activities, whereas the children of younger parents may more often be found at public, free activities. Older parents seem to have more patience and younger parents to remember how to play.

Various studies have shown that mothers today are spending more time on childrearing than did their counterparts as recently as the 1960s, despite the strong shift toward women working outside the home. More women are choosing time- and labor-intensive approaches to child care, such as reading to the child every day, preparing meals from fresh foods, and negotiating family rules rather than expecting strict obedience to a set of rules promulgated by the parents. We applaud these changes, but from personal experience we know that our stamina is not as reliable as it was at 20 and that a full day of parenting, working at a job, and performing the 85 percent of household management done by the average woman taxes our ability to stay awake and remain focused and consistent.

While your child is still an infant, establish schedules and routines. Children thrive on routine and boundaries, and so do you. It is very exhausting, to both you and the child, if he has to test your boundaries at every juncture. As soon as it is practicable, teach your child to assume small daily chores. Most children enjoy being included and are very proud to be helpful. A toddler can put an apple into a bag for your lunch when asked.

Household chores should be shared among everyone and be divided into those things that drive you crazy if they are undone and those that can wait. If you are able, hire some assistance with the ones that can wait. If you are not able to pay for help, perhaps you can do a chores swap with a friend.

Once your child is in school, you may find yourself the oldest parent at the parents' association meeting, and for a moment you may feel alien. You will soon find that mutual concern for the children outweighs any generational issues and you will have plenty of child-related matters to discuss with the young woman who could almost be your daughter. Relax.

As your child grows older, so do you, and you will be sliding into those perimenopausal years. You will tire even more easily, and your short-term memory may frighten you by failing at times when it never has before. You may be moody and feel weepy at seeing your daughter all dressed up for her grade school graduation, or angry when she starts to lash out in her own storm of hormones. Step back, talk with other women, and use whatever help you need and can get. (We think there should be someone like a doula for this stage of life, especially for women with adolescent daughters.) It is hard, but you and she will survive. Again, it is imperative that you take care of yourself. You cannot pour from an empty pitcher, nor can you take care of others when you are depleted yourself. Encourage healthy relationships between your child and other adults of whom you approve—after all, it takes a village to raise a child. Other adult role models are important to children, especially adolescents, and those people will not supplant your place in your child's heart.

Motherhood is a state of mind; your child grows up, but you will always be the mother. Even if you are in your eighties and your son in his fifties, you will worry about his health and have to restrain yourself from asking meddlesome questions. It must be biological. Letting go is a learned behavior, not a natural emotional state.

Being a parent is the hardest job anyone ever has, and the most important, and there is no school or blueprint for success. Every child will grow up with personal idiosyncrasies, and no one is perfect; it is their life journey, not yours. You are not responsible for your child's happiness. It is quite enough that you are responsible for his health and well-being as he grows up and for helping him build the tools with which to pursue his own happiness. You can do it!

APPENDIX A

Drugs and Other Substances That Are Harmful to the Fetus

Drug	Effect
ACE inhibitors	Kidney and bone defects, growth retardation
Alcoholic beverages	Growth restriction, mental retardation, facial abnormalities, small head, heart and kidney defects
Androgens (anabolic steroids, testosterone)	Virilization
Carbamazepine (Tegretol)	Brain and spinal cord defects, developmental delay, growth retardation
Cocaine	Malformations of the heart, limbs, GI tract, face, urinary tract, growth retardation, stroke
Coumadin	Bone defects, eye abnormalities, growth retardation
Lead	Miscarriage, stillbirth
Lithium	Congenital heart disease
Organic mercury (in fish)	Brain malformation, mental retardation, blindness, cerebral palsy
Phenytoin (Dilantin)	Growth retardation, mental retardation, facial defects, heart defects

Drug	Effect
Streptomycin, kanomycin	Hearing loss and damage to eighth cranial nerve
Tetracyclines	Defects of teeth and bone, staining of teeth
Thalidomide	Limb defects, heart and GI tract defects
Trimethadione, parametha-dione	Cleft lip and palate, heart defects, growth retardation, mental retardation
Valproic acid	Defects of the spinal cord and brain
Vitamin A and retinols (Accutane)	Miscarriage, central nervous system disorders, mental retardation, heart defects, cleft lip and palate, facial and eye abnormalities

Source: www.atsdr.cdc.gov/tpacts46.html or 1-888-422-8737.

APPENDIX B

Drugs and Chemicals *Not* Shown to Be Harmful to the Pregnant Woman or Fetus

acetaminophen (Tylenol)
acyclovir (Zovirax)
antiemetics (promethazine, hydroxyzine, etc.)
antihistamines (Benadryl, chlorpheniramine, etc.)
aspartame (Equal)
aspirin (but, avoid near delivery)
caffeine
chlordiazepoxide (Librium)
cleaning supplies
fluoxetine (Prozac)
hair spray
marijuana
metronidazole (Flagyl)
oral contraceptives
trimethoprim sulfamethoxazole (Bactrim, Septra)
vaginal spermicides
zidovudine (Retrovir)

Ask your doctor about any other specific drug you are taking, if you do not find it either here or in Appendix A.

APPENDIX C

Body Mass Index Table

Ht/wt	56 in	58 in	60 in	62 in	64 in	66 in	68 in	70 in	72 in
120 lb	27	25	23	22	21	19	18	17	16
130 lb	29	27	25	24	22	21	20	19	18
140 lb	31	29	27	26	24	23	21	20	19
150 lb	34	31	29	27	26	24	23	22	20
160 lb	36	34	31	29	28	26	24	23	22
170 lb	38	36	33	31	29	27	26	24	23
180 lb	40	38	35	33	31	29	27	26	24
190 lb	43	40	37	35	33	31	29	27	26
200 lb	45	42	39	37	34	32	30	29	27
210 lb	47	44	41	38	36	34	32	30	28
220 lb	49	46	43	40	38	36	34	32	30
230 lb	52	48	45	42	40	37	35	33	31
240 lb	54	50	47	44	41	39	37	35	33

Note: Reading across the top, find column closest to your height in inches. Reading down the far left column, find the line nearest your weight. In the block where height column and weight column line intersect is your body mass index.

APPENDIX D

Caffeine Content of Common Sources

Coffee	
drip	110–164 mg
percolated	99–134 mg
instant	47–68 mg
flavored, from mixes	30–60 mg
decaf	2–5 mg
Tea	
imported, brewed 5 min.	63–67 mg
American, brewed 1–5 min.	21–50 mg
oolong, brewed 1–5 min.	13–40 mg
green, brewed 1–5 min.	9–36 mg
Cola drinks	30–46 mg
Chocolate	
special dark chocolate bar	23 mg
chunk of chocolate	20 mg
candy bar	4–8 mg
cocoa mix	4–5 mg

Medications: amount should be stated on the label

APPENDIX E

Iron-rich Foods

Food	Serving Size	Iron Content (milligrams)
Meat		
Beef	4 oz	3.7
Calf's liver	3.5 oz	14.2
Lamb	1 chop	2.8
Pork	1 chop	3.9
Veal	3.5 oz	3.6
Venison	3.5 oz	3.5
Poultry		
Chicken with skin	3.5 oz	1.25
Duck	3.5 oz	2.7
Turkey	3.5 oz	1.78
Nuts		
Almonds	12–15 nuts	0.7
Brazil nuts	4 nuts	0.5
Cashews	6–8 nuts	0.6
Hazelnuts	10–12 nuts	0.5
Peanuts	1 oz	0.85
Soynuts	1 oz	1.4
Walnuts, black	8–10 halves	0.9
Seeds		
Pumpkin seeds	1 oz	3.14
Sesame seeds	1 oz	2.2
Sunflower seeds	1 oz	1.99

Food	Serving Size	Iron Content (milligrams)
Vegetables		
Beans	1/2 cup	2.7
Beet greens	3.5 oz	3.3
Broccoli	2/3 cup	0.8
Brussels sprouts	6–8	1.1
Carrots	1 large	0.7
Chard	3.5 oz	3.2
Dandelion greens	3.5 oz	3.1
Kale	3.5 oz	2.2
Mustard greens	3.5 oz	3.0
Parsley	3.5 oz	6.2
Pepper, bell	1 large	0.7
Spinach, raw	3.5 oz	3.1
Spinach, cooked	1/2 cup	2.0
Sweet potato	1 large	1.6
Turnip greens	3.5 oz	1.8
Watercress	3.5 oz	1.7

APPENDIX F

Calcium-rich Foods

Food	Serving Size	Calcium Content (milligrams)
Dairy Products (excl. cheese)		
Milk	8 oz	290
Lactaid milk with calcium	8 oz	550
Half & half	4 oz	127
Nonfat dry milk	1 oz	349
Yogurt, plain, low-fat	8 oz	415
Yogurt, plain, whole milk	8 oz	274
Cheese		
American	1 oz	175–190
Cheddar	1 oz	204
Feta	1 oz	140
Monterey Jack	1 oz	211
Mozzarella	1 oz	207
Parmesan	1 oz	355
Ricotta	1 oz	77
Swiss	1 oz	272
Seafood		
Anchovies	3 fillet	66
Bass, striped, broiled	4 oz	47
Clams	3 oz	78
Cod, dried, salted	3.5 oz	225
Crab, steamed	3 oz	84
Hake	3.5 oz	41
Herring, canned in brine	3.5 oz	147
Mackerel, canned	1/2 cup	194

Food	Serving Size	Calcium Content (milligrams)
Ocean perch	3 oz	117
Oysters, canned	3.5 oz	152
Salmon, broiled or baked	3.5 oz	414
Salmon, red, canned	2/3 cup	259
Sardines, canned in oil/brine	8 fish	354
Scallops, steamed	3.5 oz	115
Shrimp	3.5 oz	63
Smelt, canned	4–5 fish	358
Trout, brook	3.5 oz	218
Tuna, albacore	3.5 oz	26
Vegetables		
Beans	1 cup	62
Beet greens	1/2 cup	99
Broccoli	2/3 cup	88
Brussels sprouts	6–8	32
Carrots	1 large	37
Chard	1/2 cup	73
Dandelion greens	3.5 oz	187
Kale	3.5 oz	179
Mustard greens	3.5 oz	183
Parsley	3.5 oz	203
Pepper, bell	1 large	9
Pumpkin	1/2 cup	18
Spinach	3.5 oz	93
Sweet potato	1 large	72
Turnip greens	3.5 oz	246
Watercress	3.5 oz	151
Other		
Almond butter	2 tbsp	44
Brazil nuts	4 nuts	28
Hazelnuts	10–12 nuts	38
Peanut butter	1 tbsp	12

Food	Serving Size	Calcium Content (milligrams)
Pecans	12 halves	11
Soynuts	1 oz	68
Tahini	2 tbsp	128
Tofu	4 oz	258

APPENDIX G

The Loss of a Baby

This appendix should be read only if you need it. If you are currently pregnant, we advise you not to read on.

Losing a baby is devastating to a woman at any age, but for the older woman it may also represent the loss of any further hope of motherhood. In the developed world, with its modern technology and excellent health care, death of the baby during delivery or soon after birth is highly unlikely. It does happen, however, and the women who suffer this loss have a special need for emotional support.

The loss of children, both newborns and older children, used to be a common experience. Indeed, in some cultures, babies were not officially named until they had survived to age two. Thankfully, this situation has changed dramatically in the last 50 years, through advances in science, medicine, and technology. Today, the loss of a child is not a common experience.

When a newborn dies, some people, without thinking, offer simplistic responses, such as "You can have more children," or "Why don't you adopt?" These well-intentioned but unhelpful words do not speak to the grief in your heart and, indeed, for an older mother, may feel cruel. They are not intended so, but they do not help. You are grieving, and you must grieve. Those who respond helpfully will recognize this need as an appropriate response to your loss. The grieving process will help you to heal and recover. Your partner and your family will be grieving, too. Lean on each other. It seems strange that we need to validate your need to grieve for the loss of your baby, but society has become less knowledgeable about this loss as it has become increasingly uncommon.

Right after the death of a newborn, nurses on the obstetrics floor are very sympathetic and can be helpful. One of the first steps they can take is to transfer the mother from the obstetrics floor to the surgical floor, where she will not constantly hear babies crying. It is to be hoped that your hospital attendants will be sensitive to your needs: some mothers want quiet time, others need to talk out their grief.

Research shows that an important part of grieving is allowing yourself to know that your baby was a real person, by naming him or her, for example. Nurses often will offer to dress the baby in a gown and bonnet and take photos for the family. If you have photographs of your baby, we hope they provide comfort.

Societies have rituals for separating from those close to us, and for good reason—they help. You may turn to your church to conduct such a ritual. A group of your family and friends may gather to celebrate this child who has passed through your life and to offer a farewell. Expressing what is in your heart and honoring the individuality of this child whom you knew in utero is part of the grieving process.

Do not search for blame in this unfortunate event or play "what if." Accept that this child's life was nurtured by you and, though achingly brief, was meaningful.

Formal support groups begin with the obstetric units, whose nurses are trained to help you with this experience. Hospices organize and lead grief support groups. Organizations such as Compassionate Friends in the United States are specifically designed to help grieving parents. These groups understand the stages of grief, including anger, denial, and guilt, and can provide reassurance that all of these feelings are a normal part of grieving and healing.

We encourage all grieving parents to reach out for the support they need; friends and other family members can provide support in many ways and can encourage parents to make use of available resources. Professional grief counselors, psychiatrists, psychologists, social workers, and clergy can provide invaluable assistance in coping with feelings of loss. Please accept our deepest and most sincere sympathy.

APPENDIX H

Summary of Medical Tests

In this appendix, we simply reiterate the screening and diagnostic tests that are talked about in the text of this book. The purpose of this is to give you a quick and easy reference to individual tests. At the end of this appendix is a chronological listing of when the tests are usually performed.

TESTS DONE IN FERTILITY EVALUATION

Thyroid and diabetes screening.   Simple blood tests to determine whether you have a treatable medical problem that is interfering with your fertility.

Progesterone levels.   Blood test to determine whether you are ovulating; if you are ovulating, you should have a rise in your serum progesterone at day 21 of your menstrual cycle.

Prolactin levels.   Blood test for a pituitary hormone that can suppress ovulation, when present at high levels. Abnormally high prolactin levels can be caused by various drugs or by endocrine problems. If a problem is found, you will need to see either an endocrinologist or a specialist in reproductive medicine.

Pelvic ultrasound.   Examination of the outline of the uterus and ovaries using sound waves to make a picture, to look for abnormalities, and to estimate the size of the ovaries. The scan can show if you have fibroids, polyps, an abnormally shaped uterus, or other visible problems with your reproductive anatomy.

Laparoscopy.   A surgical diagnostic technique that may be used to determine the condition of your Fallopian tubes. This is an invasive test requiring general anesthetic and is not in general use in the United States, especially for older prospective mothers, who will probably be quickly referred for ART if they are not successful in conceiving without medical intervention.

Hysterosalpingogram.   An x-ray technique that is used to test the soundness of the Fallopian tubes. A dye is introduced through the cervix and then a series of x-rays follows the passage of the dye to and, if there is no obstruction, through the Fallopian tubes. This test is uncomfortable and requires some sedation and/or analgesia.

Hysteroscopy.   With a specially designed fiber-optic instrument, a doctor looks at the interior of the uterus. This test is often done in conjunction with a hysterosalpingogram (see above). The instrument is introduced through the cervix and involves a degree of discomfort similar to that caused by a hysterosalpingogram or to having an IUD placed. Sedation and/or analgesia is usually given, although anesthesia is not required.

Seminal analysis.   A specimen of semen is submitted by the male partner, produced by masturbation. The specimen must be examined in a laboratory within two hours of production, so if the man lives far from the laboratory, he may need to produce the specimen at the lab facility. Most laboratories have private spaces where this can be done. A better sample is obtained if the man abstains from sex for 3–4 days before giving the specimen.

Routine Prenatal Screening

A group of mostly blood tests is done at your first prenatal visit or when pregnancy is confirmed.

CBC (complete blood count).   A small amount of blood is drawn, from which much information can be obtained. Of particular interest is if you are anemic.

Blood glucose. This minimal screen for diabetes may be omitted if the doctor anticipates doing more precise screening later.

Blood type and Rh factor. This information is important for two reasons: first, in case you should need a blood transfusion during delivery; second, to determine whether the doctor needs to be vigilant for an incompatibility between your blood and your baby's. This incompatibility, called Rhesus disease, causes the mother's body to make antibodies against the baby—in essence, sees the baby as foreign and to be rejected. The rejection can be protected against by injections of immune globulin at appropriate times during the pregnancy.

Rubella antibody titres. This blood test measures your immunity against German measles. This is important to know, because if you are not immune, you will need to protect yourself against any exposure to people who have rubella. This can be difficult if you are a teacher or otherwise exposed to school age children, but all states require rubella immunization prior to school entry. You will be offered vaccination *after* you deliver your baby, but cannot be vaccinated while you are pregnant.

Hepatitis B antibody. Checking for this antibody shows whether you are immune to hepatitis B or might have a chronic low-grade infection that can be conveyed to your baby, even if you don't feel sick. If you do harbor this very serious illness, your baby can be given protective globulin, in addition to the routine immunization that is given to newborns.

Hepatitis C. Screening for this disease is not universally done, but it is becoming more common as the prevalence of hepatitis C rises. When it is done, it is in order to offer early counseling and treatment.

RPR (rapid plasma reagin). This test is for syphilis, a devastating illness that can be transmitted to the baby in-utero and is eminently treatable with antibiotics. If this test is positive, it is automatically confirmed by the laboratory with more specific diagnostic tests.

HIV.   Screening for HIV is viewed as a voluntary in many areas. If your doctor doesn't ask for this screening, we suggest that you request it. Babies can be protected from transmission by choice of the mode of delivery and by antiretroviral drugs. Babies are now screened at birth in all states.

PPD (purified protein derivative).   This skin test for tuberculosis is not universally applied, but many populations and geographic areas are at greater risk, for example, inner city residents, women who are occupationally exposed to patients with TB, people living on Indian reservations.

Mid-stream urine.   A frequently done test, it is used at this time primarily to check for asymptomatic urinary infection. An infection would need to be treated, to help the baby to thrive and to protect your kidneys.

Pap smear.   You are probably familiar with this cell-sampling, taken vaginally at your annual GYN checkup. It will be done at your first prenatal visit unless you have very recently had one. Although we are unlikely to aggressively treat any abnormalities until you have completed your pregnancy, it is important to know if you will need care soon afterwards. If the Pap is abnormal, you may have a colposcopy without biopsies to determine the extent of abnormal tissue and to confirm the Pap smear findings.

Chlamydia and gonorrhea smears.   These are taken at the same time as the Pap smear and are just a swabbing of your cervix with a special swab. You usually feel nothing. It is important to diagnose the presence of either of these sexually transmitted diseases because they are treatable with antibiotics and will affect the baby if not treated.

Ultrasound

Ultrasound technology is extremely helpful in pregnancy. It has given us much greater accuracy in dating pregnancies and in detecting abnormalities at an earlier stage. Ultrasound is a technique utilizing the reflection of sound waves by tissues and the conversion of those sound waves into pictures, much like x-rays. Unlike x-ray imaging, it is safe for both the mother and the baby in pregnancy and has no known risk of long-term consequences. Ultrasound scans are done at various points during pregnancy to obtain particular pieces of information.

Initial scan. Your first ultrasound will be done soon after you first visit the doctor. Its purpose is to accurately date your pregnancy. Early in pregnancy, all fetuses are about the same size per time of gestation, and this is how we can date your pregnancy.

12 weeks. An ultrasound at this time (for some women this will be the first) is done to measure the fetal nuchal translucency, measuring the layer of fluid on the baby's neck between the skin and the underlying soft tissue. This test, which screens for Down syndrome, has not yet become routine in the United States, although it is widely used in the United Kingdom and Australia.

18 weeks. An ultrasound is routinely done at 18 to 20 weeks of pregnancy, mainly to check that there are no obvious abnormalities in the baby's head, brain, face, heart, lungs, stomach, kidneys, bladder, or limbs. It is also possible at this stage to tell what the baby's gender is. Diagnosis of a problem at this stage will allow parents to either opt for termination of the pregnancy if the problem is severe and not compatible with a normal happy life or to prepare to receive a child with special needs. Some detected problems can be treated in-utero.

Other times. Ultrasounds may be done at any time in the pregnancy to elucidate problems, for example, to determine with certainty that a baby is not in the normal head first position for delivery, or to check on the development of twins. The routine ultrasounds usually tell us if the placenta is low-lying, but if you bleed during your pregnancy, an ultrasound may be done to determine the position of the placenta. One may be done later in pregnancy to determine whether there is adequate fluid surrounding the baby.

Tests for Down Syndrome

Screening Tests

Serum screening. At 15 to 16 weeks of pregnancy, blood is drawn and tested for levels of alpha-fetoprotein, estriol, human choriogonadotrophic hormone, and inhibin. These measurements are combined in a formula with the age you will be when the baby is born and a computer calculation gauges your risk of having a baby with Down syndrome or other chromosomal abnormalities.

Human choriogonadotrophic hormone and PAPP-A (pregnancy-associated plasma protein A). These are also blood tests that can be used with fetal nuchal translucency testing at 12 to 13 weeks to calculate the risk of the baby's having Down syndrome.

Screening tests, by definition, do not give a certain diagnosis; they screen for abnormalities and calculate risk. Abnormal results will lead to diagnostic tests. A normal or low risk result in these screens is not a guarantee that the baby is free of problems, but it does reassure you that significant ones are unlikely.

Diagnostic Tests

CVS (chorionic villous sampling). This test, done at 13 weeks, involves passing a needle through the cervical canal to take a sample of placental tissue. The needle is guided by ultrasound to assure good sampling and to guard against inadvertent injury of the baby. The test can also be done by an ultrasound-guided needle through the abdominal wall. The chromosomal makeup of the sampled cells can be determined within 48 to 72 hours. CVS diagnoses chromosomal abnormalities with better than 99 percent accuracy. Doing

the test at this point is important, because if there is an abnormality present and the parents want to abort the fetus, it is a relatively minor procedure at this stage of pregnancy. CVS is invasive and the woman usually requires sedation and/or analgesia. It also carries a risk of miscarriage, varying from 0.5 percent to 3 percent, depending on who does the test. The reading can be inconclusive if not enough cells are obtained to give an accurate answer or there is a difference between the placental cells and the fetal cells. The latter situation, called mosaicism, will prevent an accurate chromosomal analysis.

Amniocentesis.   This sampling of the amniotic fluid surrounding the baby is done at between 15 and 18 weeks. A long needle is passed through the abdominal wall using local anesthetic and utilizing ultrasound to guide the path of the needle. About 4 teaspoons of fluid are drawn off and sent to a lab for testing. There are two ways of examining the fluid:

A culture of the baby's shed cells can be grown and then examined for a chromosomal count. This technique gives an answer in about 2 to 3 weeks. Although this method takes some time, it gives accurate results and is the gold standard.

FISH, or fluorescent in-situ hybridization, utilizes fluorescent-labeled DNA probes that attach to specific chromosomal areas, enabling quicker identification. This method yields results in about 24 hours and is fairly accurate.

Amniocentesis, like CVS, is invasive, but it carries a lower risk of miscarriage; the risk with amniocentesis is usually no greater than 0.5 percent.

Testing for Diabetes

Screening Test

2-hour glucose tolerance test (GTT).   This test is usually done between 24 and 28 weeks, although in someone considered at higher risk (such as an American Indian or Alaskan native, a woman with a history of gestational diabetes in previous pregnancies, or someone

with a strong family history of diabetes), it may be done earlier in the pregnancy. You drink 50 gm of a sugar solution and have your blood drawn 2 hours later. A level of glucose lower than 130 mg/dL is normal. If it is higher, you will be scheduled for the 3-hour GTT.

Diagnostic Tests

3-hour glucose tolerance test.   For this test, you return to the lab fasting, and an initial blood specimen is drawn. Then you are given a 100 gm glucose test beverage to drink. Blood samples are taken 1 hour, 2 hours, and 3 hours later. These blood levels should not exceed the following values:

Fasting	95 mg/dL
Hour 1	180 mg/dL
Hour 2	155 mg/dL
Hour 3	140 mg/dL

Two or more elevated values give you a diagnosis of gestational diabetes (diabetes of pregnancy).

Two fasting blood glucose tests.   Fasting samples of blood taken on two different days both registering glucose levels of 126 or more are also considered diagnostic for gestational diabetes.

ART-Associated Test

Most of the tests associated with assisted reproductive technology (ART) have been covered above, but an important one is PGD, or preimplantation genetic diagnosis. A very few cells are taken from the developing embryo before it is implanted in the uterus. These cells are examined to be sure the normal numbers of chromosomes are present, and they can also be used to test for Down syndrome and certain other genetic conditions. If the embryo is ascertained to be abnormal, a decision can be made not to implant this particular embryo. This is an optional procedure and is not acceptable to all people.

Medical Tests and When Performed

During Fertility Workup
  Hysterosalpingogram
  Hysteroscopy
  Laparoscopy
  Progesterone
  Prolactin
  Seminal analysis

Before Implantation
  PGD

During First Trimester
  Blood type & Rh factor
  CBC
  Chlamydia & gonorrhea
  HCG & PAPP-A
  Hepatitis B antibodies
  Hepatitis C antibodies
  HIV antibodies
  Pap smear
  PPD
  RPR
  Rubella antibodies
  Thyroid
  Ultrasound
  Urine

At 12 weeks
  Fetal nuchal translucency
  Ultrasound again

At 12 to 13 weeks
  Chorionic villous sampling

At 15 to 16 weeks
  Serum screening
  Amniocentesis

At 18 weeks
  Ultrasound again

At 24 to 28 weeks
  Glucose
  HIV antibodies again

Glossary

abortion: Evacuation of the fetus from the uterus, either spontaneously or by a medical or surgical intervention, before the twenty-eighth week of gestation. Also commonly called a miscarriage.

abruptio placenta: A cause of bleeding in pregnancy or labor; when the placenta separates completely or partially from the wall of the uterus.

afterbirth: The placenta and membranes that are expelled from the uterus after the birth of the baby.

alphafetoprotein (AFP): A protein, produced first by the embryo and later by the fetal liver, which can be detected in the mother's blood and is used as a measure of fetal health.

amenorrhea: The absence of menstruation.

amniocentesis: A diagnostic procedure in which a needle is passed through the mother's abdominal wall into the uterus; through the needle, a small amount of the fluid in which the baby is floating is drawn off into a syringe. This fluid and the cells it contains are then analyzed for the presence of infection, fetal abnormalities, or genetic defects.

amnion: The layer of membrane immediately enveloping the fetus and its surrounding fluids (the amniotic fluids). Also called the amniotic sac or the "bag of waters."

amniotic fluid: The fluid surrounding the fetus in the uterus.

analgesic: Any drug that alleviates pain but does not produce unconsciousness.

anemia: A condition in which the concentration of red blood cells is lower than normal for the age and sex of the person. Because the red blood cells carry oxygen, anemia decreases the availability of oxygen to the cells of the body.

anesthetic: Any drug that produces insensibility to pain. General anesthetics produce unconsciousness and total insensibility to pain. Regional or local anesthetics produce insensibility or numbing in a particular area of the body and do not affect consciousness.

anomaly: Deviation from normal.

antibiotics: Substances that are able to destroy or inhibit the growth of bacteria that cause infection.

antibodies: Protein substances produced by the body to protect it against foreign substances, such as bacteria, viruses, or genetic material from another body.

antihistamine: A drug used to treat allergy, nausea, or vomiting. Often used for morning sickness.

anticoagulant: A drug that prevents the blood from clotting; important in the treatment of blood clots in the legs or lungs.

assisted reproductive technology (ART): A group of techniques that manipulate the sperm and egg to cause fertilization.

azoospermia: The absence of sperm, a cause of male infertility.

bearing down: The expulsive effort made by the woman in the second stage of labor.

birth canal: The vagina, the muscular passage from the uterus to the exterior.

birth control: Any of a variety of methods used to prevent pregnancy.

blastocyst: The stage of development of the embryo at the time of implantation in the wall of the uterus.

bloody show: The popular term for the expulsion of the mucus plug at the onset of labor. This is a vaginal discharge of blood-tinged mucus.

bond, bonding: An emotional attachment.

breech presentation: Bottom-first positioning of the baby in the uterus.

caffeine: A bitter alkaloid chemical present in some plants, such as tea, coffee, and cocoa. It acts as a mild stimulant to the nervous system.

cardiotocography (CTG): Simultaneous electronic monitoring of the contractions of the uterus and the baby's heart rate.

catheter: A thin plastic tube inserted in a body part for the purpose of draining or introducing fluids.

cephalic presentation: Head-first positioning of the baby in the uterus.

certified nurse midwife: A nurse who has formal training and accreditation in obstetrics.

cervix: The lower part, or neck, of the uterus, which protrudes into the vagina.

Cesarean section, C-section: A surgical birth, in which the baby is removed from the mother through an incision in the mother's abdomen and uterus. An elective, or planned, C-section is performed for medical reasons discovered before labor begins. An emergency, or nonelective, C-section is performed for unexpected medical reasons that occur during pregnancy or labor.

chlamydia: A bacterial infection that can cause infertility.

chorionic villi: Slender vascular projections from the outermost membrane surrounding the embryo. These projections enter into formation of the placenta.

chromosome: Threadlike intracellular structures that contain the DNA, or genetic material, of an individual.

colposcopy: Examination of the cervix with a telescopelike fiber-optic device in response to an abnormal Pap smear.

conception: The fertilization of an ovum by a sperm.

congenital: Present at birth.

contraception: Birth control.

deep vein thrombosis: Blood clot in the deep veins of the legs.

descent: The passage of the presenting part of the fetus through the birth canal.

diabetes: A disease in which the body cannot properly metabolize carbohydrates and sugars. Diabetes in the mother may affect the health of the baby. A woman may develop diabetes for the first time during pregnancy; this is called gestational diabetes.

dilation: The stretching open of the cervix during labor.

Down syndrome: A condition in which the baby has a chromosomal abnormality resulting in a characteristic appearance, including an epicanthic fold on the inner part of the eyelid, which gave rise to the old term for the condition, Mongolism. Usually, the person with Down syndrome has a small nose with a flat bridge and a small mouth. Down syndrome (also called Down's syndrome) is usually associated with low intelligence. The person with Down syndrome may have heart defects or other health problems.

dystocia: When a part of the baby is not able to navigate the birth canal. Shoulder dystocia is not uncommon.

eclampsia: A medical condition unique to pregnancy in which the mother develops high blood pressure, headache, convulsions; may lead to coma and death of the mother and baby.

ectopic pregnancy: Implantation of the embryo outside of the uterus, for example, in a Fallopian tube or the abdominal cavity.

EDD: Estimated date of delivery.

embolism: A blood clot that develops in the veins of the pelvis or legs and travels through the blood vessels to become lodged in vital tissue, such as the lungs (pulmonary embolism) or brain (stroke).

endocrinologist: Physician who specializes in disorders of the hormonal system, for example, thyroid problems and diabetes.

endometriosis: A condition in which tissue from the lining of the uterus grows outside the uterus, most commonly on other pelvic structures, such as the Fallopian tubes or ovaries. This condition causes pain, abnormal bleeding, and difficulty in getting pregnant.

endometrium: The lining of the uterus.

epidural: Regional anesthesia produced by introducing an anesthetic drug through a catheter into the space just outside the membrane covering the spinal cord.

episiotomy: A cut in the tissue surrounding the vagina (in the United States, usually toward the anus; elsewhere, usually to the right side), done to help with a vaginal delivery of a baby and/or to prevent tearing of these tissues.

estrogen: A hormone produced by the ovaries and the placenta. This is the "female" hormone, which is responsible for maintaining breasts and other feminine attributes, normal menstrual cycles, and normal pregnancies.

Fallopian tubes: The channels connecting the ovaries and uterus. A sperm swims up a Fallopian tube to fertilize an egg.

fetal alcohol syndrome: A condition that occurs in babies born to women who abuse alcohol early in pregnancy. It includes growth retardation, small head, characteristic facial features, mental retardation, and heart and kidney disorders.

fetal distress: The condition in which the baby's brain is not getting enough oxygen; the signs that signal this distress. Fetal distress may be mild, moderate, or severe. Most babies who suffer fetal distress recover completely when delivered in a timely fashion.

fetal monitoring: Electronic tracking of the baby's heart rate, usually done by placing an electrode on the mother's abdomen or in the skin of the baby's scalp. A read-out, or tracing, can be produced from the monitor.

fetus: The term for an unborn baby in the uterus from week eight until delivery.

fibroids: Common benign tumors located in muscle. They may be positioned just under the lining of the uterus, in the middle of the muscle wall, or just under the outer covering of the uterus.

folic acid: A B-vitamin; if deficient during early pregnancy, certain neurological problems may occur in the baby.

follicle stimulating hormone (FSH): A hormone secreted by the pituitary gland in the brain; stimulates ovulation in women and production of sperm in men.

forceps: Metal instruments, resembling barbecue tongs, which are sometimes used to assist in the vaginal delivery of a baby.

fundus: The top of the uterus.

gamete: A reproductive cell; the ovum or the sperm.

gestation: The period from conception to delivery.

gestational diabetes: See diabetes.

gravid: Pregnant.

hemoglobin: The oxygen-carrying pigment in red blood cells.

hemorrhage: Abnormal bleeding, especially heavy bleeding.

hemorrhoid: A varicose vein in or around the anus.

hormone: A chemical produced by the body, usually by a gland; it travels through the bloodstream to produce particular effects in other parts of the body.

human choriogonadotrophic hormone: A hormone produced by the developing placenta. This hormone is detected in urine and blood tests. High enough levels are present by the fourth week of pregnancy to give a positive test result.

hypertension: High blood pressure.

hypoglycemia: Low blood-sugar levels.

hysterectomy: Surgical removal of the uterus.

incision: A surgical cut.

incontinence: Inability to control the passage of urine or feces.

intravenous: Directly into a vein and thereby into the bloodstream.

in vitro: In an environment outside of the body.

labor: The coordinated sequence of involuntary contractions of the uterus that result in the birth of the infant.

lanugo: Fine, downlike hair that develops on babies in the middle of pregnancy and disappears soon after birth.

lower segment: The lower part of the uterus, located at the top of the cervix.

meconium: The dark green bowel contents of the fetus. The presence of meconium in the birth waters is a sign of fetal distress. Ordinarily, meconium is passed as the baby's feces for the first few days after birth.

membranes: The protective coverings in the body, including that surrounding the baby in the uterus. The membranes enclose the fluids that cushion the baby from trauma while it is in the womb.

midwife: A person who helps a woman in childbirth. A lay midwife has no formal obstetrical training. A certified nurse midwife is a nurse who has formal training and accreditation in obstetrics.

miscarriage: Popular term for spontaneous abortion.

morbidity: Damage or disease.

mortality: Death.

neurological: Having to do with the nervous system.

ovary: One of two almond-shaped organs located on either side of the uterus. The ovaries produce hormones and store and release eggs.

ovulation: Release of an egg (ovum) from the ovary.

ovum: Egg.

oxytocin: A hormone produced by the pituitary gland, which is located in the brain. Oxytocin stimulates the uterus to contract and the breasts to produce milk.

pelvic floor: The girdle of muscle, located inside the pelvis, which supports the pelvic organs, such as the uterus and bladder.

pelvis: The bony cage to which the hips are attached.

perinatal: During the period of time from 20 weeks of gestation to 28 days after birth.

perineum: The area of flesh between the vagina and the anus.

Pitocin: A synthetic oxytocin.

placenta: The blood-rich tissue that develops on the inner wall of the uterus during pregnancy. It is connected to the fetus through the umbilical cord and provides the fetus with oxygen and nutrients.

placenta previa: A condition in which the placenta is located, either partially or completely, low in the uterus, near or over the birth canal, such that it may tear when labor begins.

placental insufficiency: Inability of the placenta to provide adequate nutrients and oxygen to the fetus.

preeclampsia: A condition unique to pregnancy in which the mother's blood pressure rises and protein is lost into her urine.

presentation: Refers to the position of the fetus in the uterus; specifies the part of the fetus lying nearest the cervix and vagina. See breech presentation; cephalic presentation.

progesterone: A hormone produced by the ovaries and placenta.

prolapsed cord: A condition during labor or delivery in which the umbilical cord falls into the vagina, where it can be compressed, cutting off oxygen to the baby.

quickening: Faint abdominal sensation caused by movement of the fetus.

reflex: An immediate and involuntary response to a stimulus; for example, the rooting reflex of an infant.

ruptured membranes: Refers to a tear in the amniotic sac, which may occur spontaneously or because the doctor or midwife breaks the membranes for a medical reason, with the result that the waters drain out.

shoulder dystocia: Difficulty in delivering the shoulders of a baby, after the head has been successfully delivered in a vaginal delivery.

spinal anesthesia: Regional anesthesia produced by introducing an anesthetic drug through a needle into the fluid surrounding the spinal cord.

surfactant: In this context, a substance produced by the cells of the fetus's lungs after about 24 to 28 weeks, although levels may still be low at this stage of development. An adequate level of surfactant is necessary for the lungs to expand and remain open.

thrombosis: A blood clot in a vein, usually in the legs or pelvis.

toxemia: An old term for preeclampsia.

transverse lie: Position of the fetus if it is lying across the uterus horizontally.

trimester: A period of three months during pregnancy, which is divided into first, second, and third trimesters.

trisomy 21: The condition of having an extra chromosome 21. See Down syndrome.

ultrasound: A technique for obtaining an image of an internal organ or the fetus by using sound waves.

urethra: The tube from the bladder to the exterior, allowing the passage of urine.

uterus: The hollow muscular organ that sits in the pelvis between the bladder and the rectum. The fetus develops in the uterus. Also called the womb.

vacuum extractor: A traction device which attaches by suction to the head of the fetus to assist in a vaginal delivery.

vagina: The muscular passage from the uterus to the exterior of the body.

varicose: Abnormally dilated and tortuous; usually refers to veins.

ventouse: See vacuum extractor.

vulva: The fleshy lips exterior to the vaginal opening.

water: Popular name for the amniotic fluid surrounding the baby in the uterus and enclosed by membranes.

womb: Another name for the uterus.

Resources

Down Syndrome Support Groups
National Down Syndrome Society, www.ndss.org

Turner's Syndrome Support Groups
www.turnersyndrome.org

Breastfeeding
La Leche League International, 1-800-LALECHE or 847-519-7730, www.lalecheleague.org

International Board-Certified Lactation Consultants (IBCLC): Most hospital labor and delivery departments can refer you to someone local or give you contact information.

Doulas
Doulas of North America, 206-324-5440, 801-756-7331, www.dona.com

Work
www.dol.gov/esa/whd/fmla/: gives information on the federal Family and Medical Leave Act

www.workoptions.com: helpful in planning flexible work schedules

www.jobsandmoms.com: flex jobs

www.jobsharing.com

Working Mother magazine is available at many grocery stores, newsstands, and bookstores

Assisted Reproductive Technology
American Society for Reproductive Medicine, 1209 Montgomery Highway, Birmingham, AL 35216-2809, 205-978-5000, www.asrm.org

Infertility Awareness Association of Canada (IAAC), 201-396 Cooper St., Ottawa, Ontario K2P 2H7, Canada, iaac@fox.nstn.ca

International Council on Infertility Information Dissemination (INCIID), P.O. Box 6836, Arlington, VA 22206 520-544-9548, www.inciid.org

RESOLVE, 1310 Broadway, Summerville, MA 02144-1731, helpline 617-623-0744, www.resolve.org

Adoption

Adoptive Families of America, 612-535-4829
www.adoptionhelp.org
www.openadoption.org
International Families, P.O. Box 1353, St. Charles, MO 63302
National Adoption Center, 800-TO-ADOPT

Other Helpful Addresses

American Surrogacy Center, www.surrogacy.com
Center for Loss in Multiple Birth, P.O. Box 1064, Palmer, AK
    99645-1064, climb@pobox.alaska.net
Childfree Network, 6966 Sunrise Blvd., Ste. 111, Citrus Heights,
    CA 95610, 916-773-7178
Organization of Parents through Surrogacy, P.O. Box 213,
    Wheeling, IL 60090-0213, 847-394-4116, www.opts.com
Parents without Partners, 8807 Colesville Rd., Silver Spring, MD
    20910, 800-637-7074
Pregnancy hotline: a link to prenatal programs in your state,
    800-311-BABY
Stepfamily Foundation, 333 West End Ave., New York, NY 10023,
    212-877-3244
twins: www.twinsmagazine.com

Books

Cesarean Section: Understanding and Celebrating Your Baby's Birth,
    by Michele Moore and Caroline de Costa. Baltimore: Johns
    Hopkins University Press, 2003.
A Child Is Born, by Lennart Nilsson. New York: Dell Publishing,
    1965.
*Choosing Assisted Reproduction: Social, Emotional, and Ethical
    Considerations*, by Susan Cooper and Ellen Sarasohn Glazer.
    Indianapolis: Perspectives Press, 1999.
The Complete Book of Pregnancy and Childbirth, 4th ed., rev., by
    Sheila Kitzinger. New York: Knopf, 2003.
*The Complete Single Mother: Reassuring Answers to Your Most
    Challenging Concerns*, by Andrea Engber and Leah Klungness.
    Holbrook, MA: Adams Media Corp., 1995.
Creating a Life: Professional Women and the Quest for Children, by
    Sylvia Hewlett. New York: Miramax Books, 2002.
The Cultural Contradictions of Motherhood, by Sharon Hays. New
    Haven, CT: Yale University Press, 1996.
The Everything Pregnancy Fitness Book: Safe, Specially Tailored

Exercises for Before and After Delivery, by Robin Elise Weiss. Cincinnati: Adams Media Corp., 2004.

Fathering: Strengthening Your Connection with Your Children No Matter Where You Are, by Will Glennon. Conan Press, 1995.

Fathers, Sons, and Daughters: Exploring Fatherhood, Renewing the Bond, Charles Schull, ed. New York: J. P. Tarcher, 1992.

The Hidden Feelings of Motherhood: Coping with Stress, Depression, and Burnout, by Kathleen A. Kendall-Tackett, Phyllis Klaus, and Marshall H. Klaus. Oakland, CA: New Harbinger Publications, 2001.

Mayo Clinic Guide to a Healthy Pregnancy. New York: Harper Resource, 2004.

The Mother of All Pregnancy Books: The Ultimate Guide to Conception, Birth, and Everything in Between, by Ann Douglas. New York: Wiley & Sons, 2001.

New Mother's Guide to Breastfeeding, American Academy of Pediatrics, Joan Younger Meek, ed. New York: Bantam, 2002.

The Only Menopause Guide You'll Need, 2nd ed., by Michele Moore. Baltimore: Johns Hopkins University Press, 2004.

Plum magazine, from the American College of Obstetricians and Gynecologists. New York: Groundbreak Publishing, 646-201-9402, info@plummagazine.com.

A Silent Sorrow: Guidance and Support for You and Your Family, 2nd ed., by Ingrid Kohn, Perry-Lynn Moffitt, and Isabelle Wilkins. New York: Routledge, 2000.

Step by Step Yoga for Pregnancy: Essential Exercises for the Child-bearing Year, Wendy Teasdill. New York: McGraw Hill, 2000.

The Womanly Art of Breastfeeding, 7th rev. ed., La Leche League International. New York: Plume, 2004.

Women and the Work/Family Dilemma, by Judith P. Walker and Deborah J. Swiss. New York: John Wiley & Sons, 1993.

The Working Mother's Guide to Life: Strategies, Secrets, and Solutions, by Linda Mason. New York: Three Rivers Press, 2002.

Your Pregnancy Month by Month, by Clark Gillespie. New York: HarperCollins, 1998.

Index